D1713645

The
One-Hundred-Percent
Natural, Purely Organic,
Cholesterol-Free,
Megavitamin,
Low-Carbohydrate
Nutrition Hoax

THE

One-Hundred-Percent Natural, Purely Organic, Cholesterol-Free, Megavitamin, Low-Carbohydrate

NUTRITION HOAX

Dr. Elizabeth M. Whelan

Dr. Fredrick J. Stare

ATHENEUM   *New York*

1983

Library of Congress Cataloging in Publication Data

Whelan, Elizabeth M.
  The one-hundred-percent natural, purely organic, cholesterol-free, megavitamin, low-carbohydrate nutrition hoax.

  1. Nutrition. 2. Health. I. Stare, Fredrick John.
II. Title. III. Title: Nutrition hoax.
RA784.W557   1982   613.2   82-71260
ISBN 0-689-11335-8

Tables from *Cancer Facts & Figures—1982* are reprinted courtesy of American Cancer Society, Inc.

Material from *Introductory Nutrition,* ed. 4, St. Louis, 1979, by Helen Andrews Guthrie, is reprinted by permission of The C.V. Mosby Company.

To June Miller

CONTENTS

Contents

Contents

4 DIET AND HEART DISEASE: IS THERE A LINK?

Contents

CONTENTS

6 DIET AND CANCER: TAKING ADVANTAGE OF FEAR

7 SUGAR: THE KILLER ON THE BREAKFAST TABLE?

Contents

Contents

The
One-Hundred-Percent
Natural, Purely Organic,
Cholesterol-Free,
Megavitamin,
Low-Carbohydrate
Nutrition Hoax

INTRODUCTION

JUDGING FROM THE DELUGE OF NUTRITION nonsense we encounter these days, it sometimes appears that the field is slowly being converted from a science to a philosophy. What began as a systematic guide toward good health now seems, for many people, to have become a way of life.

Daily we are confronted by books, newspaper stories, magazine articles, guests on radio and television talk shows, representatives of our government agencies, and our next-door neighbors. They admonish us to eat 100 percent natural foods, avoid sugar and salt, eat more fiber and fewer eggs, consume only well-done meat (and as little of that as possible), fill up on vitamins to maintain our health, and then go on a bizarre diet to lose the excess weight we have acquired in the process. The public is understandably confused. Most of the propaganda is such a jumble of fact and fiction that even professionals have a difficult time separating the two. Occasionally, however, there are real disagreements or differences in interpretation among scientists. Public confusion on nutrition and health may have reached its peak in the spring of 1980 when, as a result of a report entitled "Toward Healthful Diets" prepared by the Food and Nutrition Board of the National Research Council, Americans saw firsthand some genuine scientific debate on the subject of dietary cholesterol, saturated fat, and heart disease.

3

Food is a highly emotional subject. It is, after all, the first known of the "creature comforts." From infancy, what goes into our stomachs is associated with love and a sense of well-being. Throughout our growing-up years the food we eat and the way we eat it is influenced by tradition, religion, habit, and cultural and social patterns. Since food is an integral part of our lives, there is little wonder it has fallen victim to so much quackery and misconception.

Faddism has always been directed at the entire spectrum of people: poor to rich, uneducated to intellectual, and young to old. For example, the famous Battle Creek Sanitarium attracted such names as Henry Ford, J. D. Rockefeller, and Harvey Firestone. The rich are obvious targets since they have money to spend. Today, many young intellectuals turn to food fads as part of a "counterculture" to our society.

It requires little intelligence for hucksters to realize that nutrition can be used to appeal to almost anyone. Thus, the general populace is being deceived needlessly by promises of magical ways to maintain health and cure diseases; to improve looks, love life (with potions more interesting than mouthwash), and social life (in ways more reasonable than switching dishwasher detergents); to increase success with higher energy levels and improved thinking ability; and to attain the Fountain of Youth, prevent crime, and overcome behavior problems. Any failure to live up to your ideal image, the faddists would have you believe, is caused by what you eat—or don't eat. For the hypochondriac, all of this is sheer delight.

Let us here interrupt with a point of fact: *Most people don't realize how easy it is to get the nutrients they need from a balanced diet.* And the ingredients of that balanced diet don't have to be purchased from any special kind of store; your local supermarket will do nicely.

Then why all the confusion? If good nutrition is that simple to achieve, doesn't it seem illogical for it to be the subject of so much conflict? It does, indeed. But a sequence of events that is becoming increasingly familiar can lead to contradictory statements even from the "experts." Here is what happens: Statements are often made on the basis of too little knowledge (or none at all). In the eagerness to generate a new theory, even a legitimate researcher may make the error of basing assumptions on preliminary data. Sometimes the data are misinterpreted, or perhaps they are not considered within the context of other relevant material. Occasionally cause and effect become reversed. We are reminded here of a talk-show host's facetious suggestion that diet drinks must cause obesity since so many fat people drink them. In that instance, of course, the statement was one of intentional humor, but the same kind of reasoning often leads to conclusions that are anything but humorous.

Since even legitimate professionals have been known to arrive at erroneous conclusions, it is easily understandable that the same can happen with consumer advocates who are usually less well trained in the scientific method. The "health-food" proponents, many of whom have had no scientific training whatsoever, carry things a step farther. They extract a fact here and a fact there, mix it with a large helping of mumbo jumbo, and feed it to the public.

Economics plays a big role. Consistently, the food industry is accused of manipulating its products in any way that will raise profits at the expense of the public's health. The barrage of criticism has caused most food processors to jump on the health bandwagon with products labeled "natural" or "additive-free."

In the meantime, the health hustlers are raking in big money from the sale of high-priced foods that are not superior to regular foods and dietary supplements that are rarely necessary. The question that immediately comes to mind is why the dollars made by the health-food industry should be more legitimate than those made by the rest of the food industry. A quick off-the-cuff answer usually has something to do with the quaint notion that the health-food-store proprietor is a "little guy," a modern-day version of the Friendly Neighborhood Grocer.

Better look again. To begin with, many such stores are part of large national chains. Between 1968 and 1973, health-food sales increased tenfold, from $60 million a year to $600 million. By 1974, Dr. Emil M. Mrak, chancellor emeritus of the University of California at Davis and chairman of a federal commission on pesticides, projected that retail sales of "organic foods" alone would reach $3 billion by 1980—and it seems that the actual figure by 1980 was even higher than that. In 1978, *New Times* carried a story on a health emporium in Los Angeles known as "Aunt Tilly's." According to the store's owners, about 2,700 people were shopping there on an average day, bringing in a daily gross of about $10,000. According to the trade magazine *Health Foods Business,* in 1979 there were 5,400 health-food stores in the United States; if individual stores within chains were counted, the number rose to 6,500. The Shaklee Corporation, one of the largest health-food sales organizations, realized sales revenues in 1981 of $454,522,000. This is not small business.

Even the government has become involved in nutrition controversies, although usually in somewhat subtler ways. Interest groups play pressure politics, and thus we see such government agencies as the Food and Drug Administration, the National Cancer Institute, and congressional committees (including the now defunct so-called "McGovern Committee") all placing a weighty thumb in the nutritional pie. But lest we give the impression that government involvement is only another term for harassment, credit should be given where due. Without such pluses as our school-lunch programs, labeling laws, additive testing, and pesticide monitoring, the American food supply could never have earned its current reputation as the most nutritious and safest in the world. The U.S. government is not trying to produce a nation of weaklings any more than the food industry—they can't afford it either!

Still, confusion perpetuates itself. Misinformation teams up with misquote. Sources echo each other until theory appears to become fact. And the more fascinating and far-out the theory, the more the media love it. Thus, sensationalism is served up as "news"—after all, who wants to hear one more rehash of the

6

Basic Four? Theory reaches the public, and the public believes.
For, they reason, there it is, right there on national television . . .
it must be true because no pseudo-nutritionist would be allowed
to say those things on the air, right?

Wrong. The First Amendment to the U.S. Constitution protects anyone's right to say—or write—anything he or she
chooses, so long as it is said without malice. Only the actual labeling of food and pharmaceutical products is controlled by law.
But while the labels cannot make false and misleading claims,
often their sellers can—and they do! Advice and sympathy are
freely available at no extra cost. The merchants and other pitch-
men are only too willing to recommend their products. Similarly,
most health-food stores are well stocked with books, magazines,
pamphlets, and all manner of other printed material spewing
forth the marvels of every conceivable "wonder" product. Unless
one is actually able to prove that a health-food peddler is prac-
ticing medicine without a license—no easy feat, but it has been
done—there is no way to prevent any of them from frightening
consumers into believing that massive changes in their diets are
needed, both to prevent and cure diseases and disorders of every
nature.

We are well aware that a controversy exists—and we are just
as aware that we are not on the most popular side. But we, too,
are frightened. We are frightened because all around us we see
the perpetration of a gigantic hoax. Some specific areas of our
concern:

1) Many consumers are falling into the trap of self-diagnosis. The danger here is twofold: People "treat" themselves
for the wrong conditions, or they employ a useless self-
treatment when what is required is legitimate medical
attention. Delay in seeking medical help can be life-
threatening.

2) Fad diets and fad eating habits can contribute to real
malnutrition.

3) Enormous amounts of vitamins, minerals, and other
dietary supplements are being consumed by people who just

don't need them. The consumer needs to know how his money is being wasted. Even more important, he needs to be made aware of the definite dangers associated with overdosing with many of these supplements.

4) Recommendations for major dietary changes do not take into account the interaction of all other nutrients. For example, although it is generally agreed that most Americans consume too many calories, primarily in the form of fat, if fat intake is reduced *too* much, undesirable nutritional changes occur. Among them is an increase in iron-deficiency anemia, because one major source of dietary fat is meat, which is also the best source of absorbable iron.

5) Money is wasted on overpriced "natural" or "organic" health-food products when equally nutritious regular groceries could be purchased at a lower price.

6) Some people have become disenchanted to a point where they don't believe *any* nutritional information.

The science of nutrition is not a collection of isolated facts; it involves the *interrelationship* of all of the fifty or so known nutrients.

Unfortunately, nutrition scientists don't have all the answers yet. But we do know that good overall nutrition is a necessary component of good health. And we know that no single nutrient or food will cure or prevent any specific disorder other than actual deficiency diseases, like scurvy or rickets. Yet the claims otherwise are rampant. As an example, less than a decade ago (years after the discovery of polio vaccine) Dr. Henry Bieler seriously proposed a causative association between polio and ice cream consumption—because the incidence of both went up in the summer. Moreover, there are no magical combinations of three or four or more ingredients that will perform miracles.

If there were such miracles, we would believe in them, too! Unfortunately, most food "miracles" are hoaxes.

Perhaps the word "hoax" requires a point of clarification. As we use the word here, we do not mean to imply that all nutritional nonsense is part of an organized conspiracy. In some cases there appears to be an undeniable intention to deceive, but for the most part the multifaceted hoax has sprung from an explosion of nutrition misinformation. The hoax has been carefully nurtured by the wishful ones looking for simple solutions—and by hucksters who are all too eager to capitalize on them.

We, and a great many other scientists, often encounter among the general public a confounding reluctance to accept the value of fact and logic. How much easier our task would be if instead we dedicated ourselves to writing something catchy like *How to Eat Crackers in Bed and Stay Slim* (subtitle: *And Improve Your Sex Life at the Same Time*). But we feel it is your right to *know* which suggestions about food and diet can improve your health, which may be potentially harmful to your health, and which are nothing more than a waste of money.

But, you may ask, why should I trust what Drs. Whelan and Stare have to say any more than I trust the other nutrition tales I hear and read? The answer is simple and straightforward: We aren't trying to sell you food products, supplements, or "miracle cures." It is not our desire to tell you specifically what to eat, or even what not to eat. *The only commodity we're pushing is common sense and nutritional "veritas," or truth.*

The ultimate victim of The One-Hundred-Percent Natural, Purely Organic, Cholesterol-Free, Megavitamin, Low-Carbohydrate Nutrition Hoax is you, the consumer. Your only weapon against nutritional and economic rip-off is an understanding of the facts as they relate to the total picture. In the pages of this book we will attempt to present and explain the scientific facts about some specific areas of nutrition and health. At the same time, we will examine some of the politics, economics, and emotion that have lent distortion to the current nutritional scene.

As you read, we ask only that you keep an open mind, realize we have nothing to sell, and that between the two of us we have reasonable professional qualifications in nutrition, medicine, and public-health education.

9

CHAPTER 1

The Nutrition
(Mis) Information
Explosion

IN THE FIELD OF NUTRITION THERE LIES A most frustrating paradox: The nutritionist untrained in journalism is generally unable to present scientific material in an entertaining style; yet the journalist untrained in nutrition is frequently able to portray his or her *un*scientific ideas in a most convincing manner. The one tends to elicit a yawn; the other a feeling of "Wow!" or at least a stirring of interest.

The public reacts with absurd judgments. While most laymen would find it unthinkable to evaluate proposed alterations for the latest missile launching, nutritional science is another matter entirely. Evidently the reasoning is that daily eating automatically invests one with a superior knowledge of food composition and metabolic processes.

What we find truly astonishing, not to mention frightening, is the extraordinary number of recipients of one or more degrees who continue to argue nutrition without fact. They expound on baseless theories; yet when asked for sources or scientific data, they have none. Either they do not know how to use, or do not wish to be bothered with, the vast stores of available scientific knowledge. A few may back their statements by citing a reference from a single textbook (which may or may not be valid), but many others are content to report what "people are saying" or "everyone knows." This kind of grapevine health lore is almost self-perpetuating.

Few people can afford—or are otherwise able—to subsist entirely on health food or homegrown products. Almost everyone indulges in some amount of "regular" food. In so doing, a great many consumers have provided themselves with a most convenient scapegoat. The most minor case of discomfort, fatigue, or social blunder can thus be attributed to whatever mysterious ingredients have been put into or taken out of the food they are being "forced" to buy and eat. The concept is simplicity itself. The marvel is that such a complete absence of logic could give birth to any concept at all, however inept. Yet there it stands—a tailor-made excuse for ignoring such *real* issues as overeating and other excesses, cigarette smoking, and personal shortcomings. How much easier to heap the blame on something vaguely known as "additives" or "processing."

Science vs. Nonscience

Scientific research can be exceedingly dull. Studies may require many years to complete. A great deal of repetition is involved, since a single study proves little or nothing. All factors must be carefully controlled, and subjects must often be ruled out at some point because of one or another interfering variable. Animal studies speed up the timing of certain investigations, but then there remains the question of how the results are to be applied to humans, since metabolic processes and biochemistry vary from species to species.

Frequently, even after years of thorough study, the results are not clear-cut, and the only conclusion is a "possible association" that "indicates a need for further study." To the scientist, such a deduction might well be an intense disappointment; among non-scientists, it isn't even likely to raise an eyebrow.

Over the years, family-oriented movies and light novels have popularized the research scientist as a rather eccentric fellow darting about in a rumpled lab coat, hair disheveled and comically oblivious to everything not connected with his current experiment. Legitimate real-life scientists are seldom so quaint. Contrary to their fictional counterparts, not only do they usually wear matching socks, but when interviewed by the press or on television, they have an almost universal tendency to speak in terms of "standard deviations," "levels of significance," and other ho-hum phrases. With rare exception, their statements tend to err on the side of caution. The presentation is generally somewhat less than lively.

FEINGOLD, PAULING, DAVIS, AND COMPANY

How much more entertaining are those persons who conjure up a startling new theory, conduct a quick study to "prove" it, and then proceed to write a book or otherwise proclaim far and wide the need for sweeping new changes in the American diet. Reader and viewer alike are treated to another fascinating "breakthrough." Never mind that it may be scientifically groundless. It's new, it's exciting, it makes wonderful conversation, and, for the most part, it's accepted with little question. Moreover, it is difficult for the average person to distinguish between a reputable nutritionist and a self-pronounced expert. Unfortunately, credentials don't always help. Two of the more recent examples here are the late Dr. Ben Feingold's work with hyperactivity (hyperkinesis) in children and his suggestion that the behavior of hyperactive children will improve if food additives, particularly colors and flavors, are removed from their diets; and Dr. Linus Pauling's comments about vitamin C as a cure for the common cold, and then influenza, cancer, and other serious ills.

Neither of these otherwise esteemed gentlemen was trained in nutrition. Dr. Feingold was an allergist. Dr. Pauling is a theoretical chemist. The latter tends to appear particularly credible since he has been twice a Nobel winner. What most of the public is unaware of is that Pauling's first Prize was awarded for his work on the nature of chemical bonds; the second was a Nobel Peace Prize for his antiwar efforts. In addition, while it is standard procedure for scientists to present the results of their research for review by specialist colleagues, neither of these doctors did so regarding their "findings" relative to nutrition. Their comments did not appear in professional journals, where they could be carefully scrutinized by nutritional scientists, rather, they were submitted directly to the popular media. Since the time of their original revelations, numerous studies by other researchers have failed to duplicate their results. But more about the theories of Drs. Feingold and Pauling in later chapters.

If one is a colorful enough character, it appears that even faulty research can be dispensed with. All that is necessary is to put together a few unrelated—and often unsubstantiated—facts, mix them with some scientific-sounding jargon, and—voila!— you can sit back and blame your tension headache on the fact that you missed your daily dose of brewer's yeast. The late Adelle Davis was a classic in this regard. Unlike most of her cohorts, Davis actually did have a smidgen of nutritional training, thus supporting the old adage about the danger of a little knowledge. In 1969, at the White House Conference on Food, Nutrition and Health, the panel on deception and misinformation proclaimed her the most damaging single source of false nutrition information in the country. And Dr. Edward Rynearson, then professor emeritus of medicine at the Mayo Clinic, said of Davis' best-selling *Let's Get Well* that it was loaded with "inaccuracies, misquotations, and unsubstantiated statements." Professor George Mann of Vanderbilt University's School of Medicine, a former colleague at Harvard's Department of Nutrition, found that mistakes in her books averaged one per page, some of them potentially lethal.

But despite these facts, Ms. Davis had a huge and adoring following. And even today her books are being sold by the thousands in bookstores throughout the country. In fact, a new book by Ms. Davis titled *Let's Stay Healthy: A Guide to Lifelong Nutrition* has recently been issued. It is interesting that although Adelle Davis died in 1974, people are still interested in keeping her misinformation alive. *Let's Stay Healthy* contains a crash course in nutrition and physiology, describing the body's needs for nutrients. It seems that this book may not be as "dangerous" as some of her other writings, but its scientific reasoning and chain of logic must, nevertheless, be questioned. Probably few of Ms. Davis' followers are aware that one of her earlier books, *Exploring Inner Space,* was penned under the name Jane Dunlap and described her many personal experiences with LSD.

But while Ms. Davis has now left her worldly shrine, her disciples live on. And they are not lonely. Just about every fallacious theory Davis missed has been thought up by someone else. Look around at your local newsstand, turn on your TV, study a few government documents, listen to the radio, browse through any bookstore. We are bombarded from all sides by nutritional misinformants. It is difficult to escape the impression that the food industry is poisoning us, the American diet is truly dismal, and what we eat is causing many of us to suffer chronic disease and premature death.

Let's take a look at some of the propaganda. Frightening or ludicrous, all of it is *scientifically unsound:*

- Gloria Swanson and her author-husband William Dufty toured the nation a few years ago to promote his book, *Sugar Blues,* claiming that America's sweet tooth is a major health problem, contributing to heart disease, cancer, and diabetes—nonsense!
- David Reuben, M.D., in *Everything You Always Wanted to Know About Nutrition,* informs us that by using modern processed foods "you are running a terrifying risk of giving yourself and your loved ones fatal cancer"—nonsense!
- In their book, *Is Low Blood Sugar Making You a Nutritional*

14

Cripple?, Ruth Adams and Frank Murray tell us that "almost 10 percent of the population is hypoglycemic" and that "hypoglycemia leads to heart disease, allergies, psoriasis, epilepsy, peptic ulcers, hyperactivity in children, asthma, multiple sclerosis, fatigue, alcoholism, and a predisposition to cancer." Their answer is a high-protein diet, eliminating sugar, starches, and caffeine; and the inclusion in the diet of brewer's yeast and supplements of zinc, chromium, and vitamins B_6 and B_{12}—nonsense!

- Nathan Pritikin, in books, articles, and literature describing his health farm, maintains that fat is the true villain in the American diet and should be almost completely eliminated. His recommendation to reduce fat to less than 10 percent of total caloric intake makes the American Heart Association guidelines look like a Roman banquet—nonsense!

- In *Killer Salt*, Marietta Whittlesey tells of the "shocking evidence linking depression, bloating, weight gain, migraine . . . and kidney disease to the salt we crave and consume— with fatal ignorance"—nonsense!

- In *Let's Eat Right to Keep Fit* (and other books), the late Adelle Davis recommended a whole collection of vitamin and mineral supplements, formulas for "balancing foods," and tips on how to discover "nature's own nutritional tranquilizers"—nonsense!

- In his books (such as *Look Younger, Feel Healthier: A Complete Guide to Better Health Through Nutrition*) and his syndicated radio program, Carlton Fredericks tells us how megavitamin therapy can treat mental disorders, how to replace nutritional elements that food packagers take out, how good nutrition prevents gynecological problems, and that "age itself is a sickness and as such can be prevented"— nonsense!

- In *Feed Your Kids Right*, Lendon Smith, M.D., tells us that "if school authorities want to stop discipline problems and vandalism in the classroom, they must do away with sugar and junk foods in the halls and close the candy stores within two miles of the school." He further states that "no teacher should be required to teach a child who did not bring his brain to school. . . Every morning each pupil should report what his breakfast contained. If he had no protein and ate mainly carbohydrates, he should be sent home." (This advice should at least afford some relief for overcrowded classrooms.) Nonsense!

- In *The Natural Way to Health and Beauty,* model Toni De-Marco warns against drinking any liquids or eating fruits within thirty minutes before or after a meal to avoid diluting one's digestive juices. She also tells us she has "heard" that chocolate takes two weeks to digest and recommends a partial fast as a means of "beginning a cure for every illness there is." This book is jam-packed with other preposterous gibberish, but perhaps none is more absurd than the following: "Even though the stomach has two compartments and can usually separate foods with opposing digestive requirements, it sometimes cannot separate certain fruit and vegetable mixtures which consequently sour and contaminate the bloodstream." (Even a failing elementary-school student is likely to know that the human stomach has only one "compartment," and the sentence topples downhill from there. Perhaps Ms. DeMarco is presenting her material for cows, which, in order to "chew their cuds," do possess a compartmentalized stomach, but they have four compartments, not two!) Nonsense!

- *Dr. Frank's No-Aging Diet* claims to be the first diet book based on the scientific breakthrough of our age: the discovery of the "double helix." Through a diet enriched with the nucleic acids RNA and DNA, he tells us, every cell in our bodies can be young again. His inevitable corollary is that such a diet will help prevent or suppress the degenerative diseases common among older persons (such as heart disease, arthritis, and adult-onset diabetes). On page 12, Frank admits that his theory has not been proved, but he blithely carries on, for 143 more pages, on the grounds that it also has not been *dis*proved. The bottom line on his recommendations is to eat more sardines—nonsense!

- In *Bee Pollen and Your Health,* Carlson Wade presents "new material explaining what bee pollen is, how it has helped in the treatment of illness, how it has helped bring ordinary athletes up to championship performances"—nonsense!

- In *Everything You've Always Wanted to Know About Energy But Were Too Weak to Ask,* Naura Hayden tells us that the true energy food is protein, and that sugar gives us energy for only about ten minutes. She goes on to explain that the real problem with sugar is that it burns up all the B vitamins in our systems in order to be metabolized, and that those missing B "vites" (as she calls them) can leave us "very jittery, anxious, and tense, and can cause canker sores, ulcers, heart attacks, acne and deep psychiatric depressions." The back-cover blurb quotes Dr. Robert Atkins, of the *Dr. Atkins' Superenergy Diet,* as saying Hayden's advice "can give us the kind of energy that will make us all superstars"—nonsense!

- In *Orthomolecular Nutrition,* Abram Hoffer and Morton Walker explain "how the seemingly inevitable diabetes, cancer, heart disease, ulcers and hypoglycemia, with related mental illness, can be prevented by optimum diet, with proper vitamin and mineral supplementation"—nonsense!

- In *Stay Young Longer,* Linda Clark expounds on the remarkable powers of lecithin. To mention just a few of its alleged wonders, lecithin supposedly: reduces cholesterol in the blood and dissolves the plaques of atherosclerosis; acts as a brain food and keeps older people more alert; helps fight acne; softens aging skin; acts as a tranquilizer; restores sexual powers; redistributes weight, shifting it from unwanted parts to parts where it is needed; prevents and cures fatty liver; and, with the help of vitamin E, lowers insulin requirements in diabetics—nonsense!

- In *Folk Medicine: A Vermont Doctor's Guide to Good Health,* the late Dr. D. C. Jarvis relies on honey and apple-cider vinegar, either alone or in combination, to cure almost everything. Although this book was first published in 1958, it continued as a best-seller into the sixties and, in paperback form, is still on the shelves of most bookstores. A tablespoon of honey, Jarvis tells us, will cure many migraine headaches within half an hour. (If it doesn't, take another tablespoon.) His advice for the overweight is to take two teaspoons of vinegar in a glass of water at each meal. This, he alleges, makes it possible "to burn the fat in the body instead of storing it." A single teaspoon of vinegar in water will prevent morning sickness, and a vinegar/honey mixture will increase fertility. This book is a medicine man's dream. (We would like to note here that the original publication lists Jarvis as a member of the Academy of Opthalmology and Otolaryngology, indicating that he is an "eye, ear, nose, and throat" specialist—not a nutritionist.) Nonsense!

- Nutrition articles appear continuously in women's magazines. One issue of *Family Circle,* for instance, carried an article which offered vitamin formulas to protect against dandruff, balding, wrinkles, and other symptoms of aging; as well as "informing" us that niacin guards against bad breath and that a B_{12} deficiency can cause body odor. Space permits only this single example, but others are far from scarce. The nearest newsstand will likely be supplied with more than you are willing to read—about such nonsense!

- In *Jane Brody's Nutrition Book,* the *New York Times* personal-health columnist presents a typical media viewpoint on the current status of nutrition in America. While some parts of the book are sensible and accurate, the author's simplified interpretations of nutrition research result in misleading advice to her readers. According to Brody, the modern guide to healthful eating includes variety, moderation, and evolutionary change. True; yet, in her book, processed foods, packaged products, additives, and food technology are all condemned (nonsense!), while Grandma's cooking and the old ways of eating are supported. Readers are therefore advised to avoid—rather than be moderate in their intake of—many of the modern food products currently available, which limits dietary variety and certainly puts a halt to dietary evolution.

• As if worrying about your own nutrition weren't enough, in *The Healthy Cat and Dog Cook Book,* Joan Harper tells us we also need to worry about our pets' diets. She recommends regular supplements of brewer's yeast, cod-liver oil ("pets love it"), wheat germ, vitamin E, alfalfa meal, kelp powder, Epsom salts, lecithin, bran, zinc, and apple-cider vinegar. This last, she claims, "has helped to relieve arthritis in both people and animals," and since a teaspoon in a pint of drinking water has supposedly been shown to keep goats free of worms and lice, "it might do the same for dogs"— nonsense!

The specific messages we receive about "dangerous" chemicals in our food are just as plentiful. A number of the preceding sources have sounded the alarm, but we include here a few additional examples:

• As mentioned earlier, the late Dr. Ben Feingold in *Why Your Child Is Hyperactive* claimed that behavior disturbances and learning disabilities are caused by the presence of artificial food flavors and colors—nonsense!

• Beatrice Trum Hunter in *The Great Nutrition Robbery* warns that "the FDA encourages the manufacture of imitation foods" and maintains that the health of Americans is being threatened by cancer-causing agents in our diet— nonsense!

• Marian Burros in *Pure and Simple* presents "delicious recipes for additive-free cooking." The implicit premise of the book is that natural foods are better and safer. Thus, it offers "up-to-date advice on avoiding ingredients that contain chemicals"—nonsense!

• In *The Prevention of Incurable Disease,* Dr. M. Bircher-

Benner, now deceased, taught that "incurable disease is always 'unnatural' and that its root cause is faulty nutrition—a diet overloaded with animal protein and poisoned with additives, which rob the body of its natural defenses"—nonsense!

• In *Beware of the Food You Eat,* by Ruth Winter, the publisher (Signet) asks, "Have you had your poisons today?"—a query that has since inspired the creation of numerous cartoons—nonsense!

• *Prevention Magazine,* which now claims a circulation of over three million, regularly speaks of the "poisons" in our food and yearns for a return to the 100 percent natural way of life. A recent article condemned government regulatory agencies for negligence, noting that "the FDA wants us to turn in our brains"—nonsense!

• Speaking of food additives, David Reuben, M.D., writes: "The major food companies have launched a massive campaign against the Delaney Clause because they like to put things in your food that cause cancer"—nonsense!

• In *Eater's Digest,* Dr. Michael F. Jacobson, a microbiologist and self-appointed nutritionist and "consumer advocate," sums up his case against food additives this way: "Some food additives make foods safer, others make foods cheaper, others make foods more or less nutritious; all food additives help companies make money, and that, in a nutshell, is why additives are usually used"—nonsense!

Claims that the American diet is life-threatening and that there are carcinogens in our food supply are not limited to books and magazines. Consider what has been happening in the federal government:

• In March 1977, the Food and Drug Administration (FDA) proposed a ban on saccharin, then our only available artificial sweetener, asserting that it caused cancer in animals and might present a threat to human beings. Yet the claim that it caused cancer in animals was based on a single study. Seventeen other animal studies failed to reach the same conclusion.

- The U.S. Department of Agriculture (USDA) and the FDA expressed concern in the late 1970s that the presence of nitrites in cured-meat products might threaten our health. Yet nitrite in these products actually protects health by preventing the growth of dangerous bacteria. Additionally, the government rarely mentions that most of our nitrite intake comes from natural sources, including many vegetables and drinking water. Nitrite recently became the subject of a remarkable federal flip-flop. In August 1978, FDA and USDA announced that sodium nitrite would be banned as a food additive, after a gradual phaseout. This action was prompted by the results of a rat study, performed under contract to FDA, which seemed to indicate that nitrite had caused lymphoma, a type of cancer, in the animals.

  The federal agencies seemed very sure that nitrite caused cancer; sure enough to publicize this alleged hazard widely and to plan a phaseout that would have had drastic effects on meat producers and consumers. Yet, two years later, in August 1980, all plans for the nitrite phaseout were dropped. Why? A reexamination of the *same* rat data by independent experts showed that nitrite hadn't caused cancer in the animals, after all.

- The Senate Select Committee on Nutrition and Human Needs, chaired by Senator George McGovern, told us in a 1977 report that we were in the midst of an epidemic of noninfectious "killer disease" (their words, not ours). The McGovern Committee (which, it should be noted, was a legislative rather than a scientific body) proposed a drastic restructuring of the American diet and strongly suggested that major improvements in the nation's health would result if its recommendations were carried out.

  The Committee's recommendations were published as the Dietary Goals for the United States. The goals (outlined on the list below) called for a substantial reduction in dietary fat (from 42 percent of the calories in our current diet to 30 percent) and a reduction in the proportion of this fat that is saturated. They also called for a substantial increase in carbohydrate intake (from 46 percent of the calories in our current diet to 58 percent). This increase should come entirely from a drastic increase in intake of complex carbohydrates (starches), since the goals also called for a *reduction* of the other type of carbohydrate in our diets, sugar.

The goals also called for (not shown on the list) calorie control to avoid overweight, a reduction in cholesterol consumption to 300 mg per day, and a reduction in salt consumption.

How would people be expected to eat in order to meet

THE AMERICAN DIET

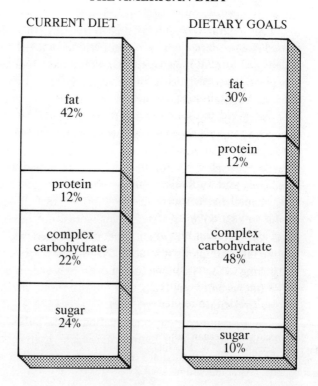

CURRENT DIET — fat 42%, protein 12%, complex carbohydrate 22%, sugar 24%

DIETARY GOALS — fat 30%, protein 12%, complex carbohydrate 48%, sugar 10%

these goals? A marked reduction in the use of sugar and sugar-rich foods, salt and foods high in salt, butter and whole milk dairy products, eggs, meat, and foods high in fat would be necessary. Consumption of whole grains, fruits and vegetables, poultry, fish, and unsaturated fats would have to increase to make up the difference.

Clearly, implementation of the goals would involve major changes in the eating habits of most Americans. As we will show later in this book, some of the goals advocated by the McGovern Committee are not backed up by substantial scientific evidence, and some of the proposed dietary changes may not be necessary or even desirable.*

- In the summer of 1979 the Surgeon General's report, *Healthy People,* recommended essentially the same guidelines as the McGovern report; and in early 1980 the Department of Health, Education and Welfare and the Department of Agriculture released their long-awaited *Dietary Guidelines for Americans.* In twenty pages of expensive multicolor printing, this pamphlet suggests that we all should:

    1) Eat a variety of foods
    2) Maintain ideal weight
    3) Avoid too much fat, saturated fat, and cholesterol
    4) Eat foods with adequate starch and fiber
    5) Avoid too much sugar
    6) Avoid too much sodium
    7) If you drink alcohol, do so in moderation

    As we shall show, some of this advice is unnecessary. The rest is so vaguely worded as to be of little use. After all, one man's moderation may be another man's orgy.

- Dr. Arthur Upton, then director of the National Cancer Institute, recently recommended that Americans modify their diets (in the same general direction as Senator McGovern recommended) to reduce our risks of developing cancer. Yet

---

* Apparently the Reagan Administration recognizes this. Assistant Secretary of Agriculture C. W. McMillan now states that nutrition information offered by the government now and in the future will be based "on fact and not opinion." As of this writing, the "goals" are drifting into oblivion.

scientists don't even agree on whether or not enough is known about diet/cancer relationships to justify *any* dietary recommendations. Yes, this despite the 1982 report of the National Academy of Science!

- In the mid-1970s the Federal Trade Commission, concerned about "junk foods" undermining the nutrition of American children, recommended that advertising of certain foods on television be prohibited during children's viewing hours. Yet there is no reason to believe that these foods are harming our children's health. Fortunately, in 1981 the FTC took the same viewpoint and dropped their recommendation concerning TV advertising for children.
- The Department of Agriculture has proposed that the sale of "minimal nutrition foods" in schools be prohibited, the premise again being that soda, candy, and snack foods have caused a major nutrition problem in children.

The nutrition advice showered on us from all sides is certainly not limited to discussions of overall diet or the additives it contains. A favorite specialty area is weight control. So many publications deal with this topic that an uninformed dieter setting out to shed a few pounds must surely have difficulty in deciding how to go about it. In chapter 3 (on obesity), we will describe a number of these reducing diets and point out the hazards involved. Many weight-loss methods are downright dangerous, most notably those advising the elimination of all dietary fats or carbohydrates—or all solid food. But just as many others advocate a wide variety of useless gimmicks, from special supplements and "wonder" foods (like bran or grapefruit) to hormone shots and reducing-pajamas.

That the term *nonscience* sounds very like the term *nonsense* is probably no accident.

The Evolution of Confusion

Why so many authors (most of whom have no professional qualifications in nutrition), government agencies, and even a few credentialed scientists make the kinds of ill-founded claims we have just mentioned is partly a matter of speculation, but a few points are patently obvious. Anyone who pays the least attention to politics is aware of a certain degree of fraternalism between government and various public-interest groups. To ignore powerful lobbyists is to lose votes.

Inevitably, personalities come into play—and that principle applies whether we are speaking of the self-styled pseudo-expert searching for a power base or the politician taking an ego trip.

The power struggle within the federal government itself has grown into what has been described on more than one occasion as a "turf war." The National Institutes of Health, as an arm of Health and Human Services (HHS) has been conducting nutrition research for many years. The National Institute on Aging (and its predecessor agency) alone has studied nutrition in several thousand persons for over two decades. Yet in 1977, Congress named the Department of Agriculture "lead agency" in nutrition research. Consequently, there has been a good deal of mudslinging between HHS and USDA. While this dual involvement could lead to a certain amount of healthy competition, unavoidably it must also lead to a certain amount of wasteful duplication of effort. Again in 1981, human nutrition was downgraded in the Department of Agriculture, and control may gravitate back to HHS, or, for those in the inner circles, H_2S.

To be sure, the sweet smell of money plays a key role. In mid-1979, $170 million was the projected amount to be spent during that year for human nutrition research by the USDA and HEW combined. That figure was up from $50 million spent in 1977 by the entire U.S. government. To quote Daniel S. Greenberg's interpretation in *The New England Journal of Medicine* (2/28/80): "The issue isn't nutrition research; rather, it's the division of money and power to do the research, plus the influence over public policy that comes from setting priorities and managing information." In June of 1979, William J. Broad of the American Association for the Advancement of Science counted fourteen congressional committees and twenty subcommittees looking into national nutritional needs. He also mentioned that "there are now fourteen agencies under seven different departments involved in human nutrition research." That's a lot of division of money and power.

Perhaps the real wonder is that the conglomeration hasn't yet collapsed into total chaos.

The health-food industry isn't exactly losing money either. Its success was nicely summed up in a *Newsweek* article entitled "Diet Crazes" (12/19/77): "The major difference between organic foods and the ones available at the supermarket, conclude most experts, is that they cost about twice as much." And that doesn't even touch on the extremely healthy markup on most dietary supplements.

And what of the economic pursuits of some of the individual would-be nutritionists? Without their personal tax returns at our fingertips, we have to rely on a certain amount of estimation. Nevertheless, the estimates for the author we shall here use as an example are exceedingly well calculated and, if anything, conservative. (We thank Ronald M. Deutsch, author of *The New Nuts Among the Berries* and other excellent books, for supplying some of the figures.)

Our example, typical of many others, is Dr. Robert C. Atkins. In its first year alone, *Dr. Atkins' Diet Revolution* sold some 1,100,000 hardcover copies. Assuming that Atkins received the usual 15 percent royalty (based on the retail price), his own take works out to $1.04 per book—a total of $1,144,000 for one book during one year. After nineteen printings in hardcover by David McKay, in 1973 Bantam began publishing the book in paperback and by May 1979 had completed an additional 32 printings. Of course, paperbacks don't net quite as much income for the authors, usually a mere 10 percent of the retail price (25 cents per copy in this case), but this was augmented somewhat by fees for condensations of the book that appeared in both *Cosmopolitan* and *Woman's Day*. During this time, Atkins continued his very lucrative private medical practice. He was quoted in a *Women's Wear Daily* interview as saying that he and his partner were treating approximately 500 patients a week.

Despite an enormous amount of criticism by the American Medical Association and numerous individual authorities, *Diet Revolution* still appears in the bookstores, and would-be dieters are still being lured by its promise of being "the high-calorie way to stay thin forever." And, in 1977, Crown was only too eager to publish *Dr. Atkins' Superenergy Diet* (a condensed version of which appeared in *Family Circle*). And why not? McKay, the publisher of Atkins' earlier book, would have made an estimated gross of $4.5 million for *Diet Revolution* during its first year of sales. For that kind of income, the publishing business is not too likely to concern itself with the possibility that its products might be based on misinformation and false premise. Author Ronald Deutsch, whom we mentioned before, puts it very well: "Even on a much more modest scale, a diet or health-food book remains a good investment. . . . It is hard to find a distinguished publisher which has not given us an undistinguished book on nutrition."

Nevertheless, we would be remiss if we did not also mention that a few writers and other promoters of pseudo-nutrition do seem to ring a note of sincerity. This is most evident in some of those theories that are based on folk medicine or religious dogma. But almost invariably, their "information" is actually misinformation because it is based on too much premature evidence and/or too little real knowledge.

Even more disheartening are those works that avoid the real issues at stake. Individuals and groups of all description show a tendency to get carried away with the possible link between diet and heart disease, for instance, while ignoring other facts already in evidence, such as the association between smoking and heart disease. In other words, as we will discuss more fully in succeeding chapters, we need to concentrate a great deal more on what we *do* know and concern ourselves a bit less with what is not yet proven reality.

"'REVOLUTIONARY'' MAGIC

Every once in a while the argument is raised that perhaps many far-out theories really do work, but that scientists have not yet been able to unlock their secrets. The reality is that most of the popular theories being touted today are anything but new. Apple-cider vinegar, for instance, has been a popular folk remedy for centuries. Its reputed medicinal powers have been numerous, and at one period in America's history it was even used in attempts to cure yellow fever.

One of the earliest recorded miracle foods dates back to the second century B.C., when Cato wrote of the wondrous powers of cabbage. The Romans considered it a cure-all, and while it was hardly that, it often did restore health to the sick. The reason? Scurvy, an ailment caused by vitamin C deficiency, was common at the time, and cabbage is a good source of vitamin C. Thus, anyone suffering from scurvy did indeed become "magically" cured by regular consumption of cabbage. What is less understandable is why today cabbage again commands a similar mystical reputation in certain circles. (Adolphus Hohensee and others have recommended cabbage juice to cure ulcers, for instance.)

Undoubtedly, the biggest and most enduring boondoggle of all is the sale of seawater. The idea is that since all life originally came from the sea, the sea and its products offer the key to good health and a long life. According to Dr. James Harvey Young in *The Toadstool Millionaires*, that particular form of quackery in this country dates back to 1630. A mere ten years after the Pilgrims arrived, a resident of the Massachusetts Bay Colony was fined five pounds for peddling "a water of no worth nor value" as a cure for scurvy. It was bottled Atlantic Ocean. And that was only the beginning.

By the 1920s, the Pacific Ocean apparently became more popular. A wealth of products appeared, often with such cleverly worded claims that they violated no law and remained for many years on the market. An example is one called Cur-O-Sea, which was described as "one of the most glorious manifestations" of the "one healer ... Nature." The family size sold for five dollars a gallon. For the economy-minded there was Zola the Wonder Water, a dehydrated (!) version advertised as "concentrated water." For only one dollar the buyer could purchase enough of a white powder to make twenty-five to forty gallons of seawater.

The powder was actually about a nickel's worth of Epsom salts, which was a pretty good markup considering the low overhead. But still another product turned out to be only tap water, which must have realized even greater profits.

And today? Logic continues to be more prevalent among the sellers than the buyers. In the late 1970s, Sears Roebuck began opening health-food departments in some of their retail stores. One in California, less than ten miles from the ocean, offered Pacific Ocean water at $1.95 a pint. (Inflation is everywhere.) Of course, this brand has the added advantage of having been filtered, which must account for its high cost.

Health-food stores and mail-order houses throughout the country do a continually thriving business on sales of sea salt, kelp, and "organic ocean fish" ("from the pollution-free waters of the Atlantic," one store sign read). The bottom line on all this is that there is *nothing whatsoever* in seawater—or sea salt or seaweed—that is not readily available in the foods we commonly eat as part of a balanced diet based on the Basic Four Food Groups. But the sea does indeed have one health-giving property: it strengthens the bank accounts of its profiteers.

BATTLE CREEK OR BATTLEGROUND?

Historically, many of the lead characters in America's nutrition drama did not set out to achieve wealth. That some of them were eventually able to cash in on their wild theories was almost accidental. And, unquestionably, they all enjoyed the power bestowed on them by their followers.

Generally, the theories began with one or two valid health principles—for instance, the use of whole-grain rather than white flour which, before nutrient fortification of flour became customary, made good nutritional sense. But the basic premise invariably was carried to an extreme and became hopelessly entangled with religious and personal beliefs. "Naturalists" of today would be appalled to find that their predecessors believed their daily doses of bran would be of value only if accompanied by such other habits as cold baths, enemas, and sexual abstinence.

One of the earliest of the bran worshipers was Sylvester Graham, who preached the fear of eating the wrong food along with the fear of God. Graham decided early that, like the apes, man's natural food must be vegetable, and he insisted that eating meat resulted in vile tempers and sexual excesses. The latter in turn led to insanity, he ranted to the multitudes, a notion that found good company in such other absurdities as his assertions that tea caused delirium tremens, chicken pie caused cholera, and that the ultimate salvation for sinners was Graham flour. His namesake cracker has survived for a century and a half.

In 1876, Dr. John Harvey Kellogg, in conjunction with a group of Seventh Day Adventists headed by Sister Ellen White, opened what was probably the nation's first health center. Located in Battle Creek, Michigan, the chic sanitarium afforded a superb place for Kellogg to experiment with his endless screwball ideas. He was very selective about his patients, though, refusing to accept anyone who wasn't going to get well. Kellogg eventually created the first dry cereals, and his cornflakes carried him to fame and riches, hardly in keeping with the simple beliefs of the Adventists. Sister White stamped her saintly foot and a schism erupted, but, undaunted, Kellogg maintained his power and success minus the blessings of the church. Like so many of his colleagues, the older he grew the more eccentric his ideas became. He insisted that poisoned intestines were the real cause of all disease and that hot food caused cancer. For high blood pressure he advocated strawberries or grapes—in amounts that varied between ten and fourteen pounds a day. And so on.

Enter C. W. Post, and the corporate scrimmage of the cereal magnates began. The feisty Post violently opposed many of Kellogg's ideas, with good reason, but his own were no improvement. In 1898, an ad for Grape Nuts (one of the early Post successes) claimed to cure appendicitis, tuberculosis, and malaria; feed the brain and tighten loose teeth. For years Battle Creek thrived as a center of absurdity.

At about this same time, Horace Fletcher read about British statesman William Gladstone's reasoning that since man has thirty-two teeth, the food he eats should be chewed thirty-two times. Fletcher, taking that one a step further, decided that man would do even better if he chewed each mouthful fifty to sixty times. His idea had something to do with enabling the chewer to better explore his taste sensations, but more importantly, food wastes would be prevented from accumulating in the intestines and thus causing sickness. "Fletcherizing" became a byword in countless households and was a standard part of the treatment in Kellogg's sanitarium. Eventually, Fletcher arrived at the conclusion that if well-chewed food kept the body's digestive system clean, no food at all would keep it even cleaner. He began to advocate fasting, often for several days at a time, and told a prominent women's magazine of the day that fasting would lead to less work for the housewife, as well as being a boon for the food budget. All that mastication probably resulted in such exhausted jaws that occasional fasting was a relief.

(Some of our older readers may recall being treated to Fletcher's Castoria for childhood constipation problems. Promising to neatly scour out little systems, its trademark slogan was "Babies Cry for It." Hmmph.)

BODY BEAUTIFUL

At the end of the nineteenth century, along came Bernarr MacFadden and the beginning of the physical-culture movement. MacFadden was dearly proud of his overdeveloped muscles and earned his early reputation by posing with as many of them exposed as the law would allow. Perhaps the most notable fact about MacFadden is that he was the first of the health quacks to use mass media techniques in promoting his nutrition and other health misinformation. It was simple enough. By the 1920s, he had launched a publishing empire which included such magazines as *True Story, True Romances, True Detective,* and others. MacFadden was perhaps the first in a long series to advocate grapes as a cure for cancer. His prescription was a few days' fast, followed by eating as many grapes as the victim could hold. He was even audacious enough to offer $10,000 to anyone who could prove that grapes would *not* cure cancer.

31

Somewhere in the 1920s, the morass of nutritional hogwash began piling still higher with the inspirations of Gayelord Hauser. His notions about special foods to promote good looks became immensely popular with Hollywood stars, as well as beauty seekers everywhere. Among his favorites were skim milk, brewer's yeast, and wheat germ. In one of his books, *Look Younger, Live Longer,* Hauser revived the centuries-old wonder ingredient, blackstrap molasses. "Living foods for a living body" was his motto. Hauser's "beauty bars" and propaganda still dominate the market in the worlds of both health food and fashion.

THE CIRCLE CLOSES

By the 1940s, another "lord," in the person of Lelord Kordel, had arrived on the scene. His major claims were that rare meat and honey would cure everything from rheumatism to heart disease, and that they would prevent aging, premature death, and loss of sexual ability. Thus, we have run the gamut in the meat department: from the recommendation of none at all to one which required that meat be barely cooked through, a procedure that was not entirely safe during those years.

There have been so many other faddist personalities that one could play pick-a-theory with the greatest of ease. Dr. Jarvis, the Vermont folk-medicine proponent already mentioned, alleged that alkalinity in the body was a threat to American health, and that acidity could be increased by avoiding such foods as white sugar and citrus fruits, and preceding each meal with—of course—a couple of tablespoons of apple-cider vinegar. In direct contrast, during the early 1900s, journalist Alfred Watterson McCann insisted that *acidity,* resulting from refined foods including sugar, drew "lime salts" out of the muscles and thereby contributed to disease. So here we have refined sugar causing either acidosis or alkalosis, whichever you prefer. (McCann's employer, the *New York Globe,* had even provided him with a little room and a white coat so that his health articles could legitimately carry the words "tested in my lab." For whatever reason, he is still known today as a "pure food" crusader.)

Similarly, a few decades ago word got around that milk was a cause of cancer. On the other hand, the late Adelle Davis urged everyone to drink a quart of milk every day to *prevent* cancer. Since she eventually succumbed to that very disease, some other health-food guru is inevitably destined to revive the milk-causes-cancer theory.

Ad infinitum. It all depends on what or whom you choose to believe. Whatever favorite theories you yourself may have fallen heir to, someone out there in healthfoodland is sure to back you up—and someone else will be happy to "prove" you wrong. The confusion perpetuates itself.

A Success Story: The Health Faddists

While it will seem improbable to at least some readers that the nutritional fictions of past generations should continue to persist, the truth is that a great many of them do. The growth in knowledge of both nutrition and the causation of disease (or, in some cases, an awareness of the current *lack* of knowledge) has provided fertile territory for an accompanying growth of flummery. The misapplication of isolated facts, coupled with myths and half-truths dredged up from the past, has led to a hyperadulterated nutritional hodgepodge.

During this century, scientists learned that a number of diseases were caused by vitamin or mineral deficiencies. These genuine associations are now fairly common knowledge: scurvy and vitamin C; beriberi and certain of the B vitamins; rickets and vitamin D; iron-deficiency anemia and iron; goiter and iodide. But from these associations, many have drawn the erroneous conclusion that most other disorders are also food-related. It's easy enough to see how much of this evolves, even semiconsciously. If, for instance, your grandmother always told you that lemonade (which contains a small amount of vitamin C) was good for colds, and now Linus Pauling is telling you that vitamin C is good for colds, it might hardly seem fitting to argue with both of these higher authorities. Your assumption of truth may be only casual or subconscious, but it is there, nevertheless. Unlike Pauling's megadosing proposals, Grandmother's lemonade was harmless, and (sweetened with honey, of course) it probably tasted good.

MOTHER NATURE'S FAMILY TREE

Obviously, it is not entirely as simple as all that. The naturalist movement of the past several years has caused many manufacturers and consumers alike to climb on the back-to-nature bandwagon. Ever since the publication of Rachel Carson's *Silent Spring*, environmentalists have been clamoring about the misuse of pesticides, in some cases with due cause. But a large part of the naturalist crusade launched by the younger generation was not so much proenvironment as it was an antiestablishment gesture. The idea was to abandon modern technology and return to "living off the land," an admirable endeavor for those who live in agreeable parts of the country and who have the time to carry out such pursuits. But as often as not, the enthusiasm of the nature people is not matched by food production in the backyard or communal garden, and many soon find themselves augmenting their diets with superfoods from the nearest health-food store—all "natural," of course.

The youth cult grew. Inevitably. As stories floated around about the possible carcinogenic effects of almost everything, people began to wonder. Perhaps, they pondered, the junior citizenry really did have the right answer. And, too, who among us wouldn't like to remain forever young? Maybe nature did indeed hold the key.

Just as inevitably, the health-food hucksters and vitamin companies were quick to cash in on the trend. All kinds of natural remedies tempted buyers to rid themselves forever of gray hair, wrinkles, age spots, baldness, middle-age spread, and sex problems. The elderly were promised revitalization, and the young were assured they would keep looking that way (or better). Everything from headaches to heart disease, people were told, could be prevented with vitamin supplements, the right wonder foods, and "organically" grown produce. Shoppers were cajoled into paying twice as much money for scabby "organic" apples they would have scoffed at in a supermarket—and they were even happy about it.

The "regular" food industry also began to use this marketing ploy to promote sales. "Nothing artificial" began appearing on the labels of more and more products. The cosmetic industry rapidly followed suit, and thus we were treated to cucumber face cream, strawberry soap, and balsam shampoo; all pH-regulated, created from natural ingredients, and fortified with protein. From there, the situation grew ever more ludicrous. One manufacturer put out a natural deodorant, and still another advertised natural cookware. One season, Saks Fifth Avenue introduced a line of natural clothes. (No, they weren't fig leaves; in fact, they rather closely resembled other, presumably unnatural, clothes of the day.)

The physical-culture movement, although not new, was given a considerable boost by John F. Kennedy during the time he was President. For a great many sedentary Americans, a new focus on exercise was a very good thing. In moderate amounts and with some frequency, it will contribute to weight control, heart health, improved muscle tone, and a feeling of well-being. But here again the physical-fitness experts (or pseudo-experts) had their hands out. Jack La Lanne became a household word, and health centers sprang up everywhere. Most included health bars that served up such delicacies as celery-juice cocktails and Tiger's Milk, as well as enticingly named house specialties.

In addition to a physical culturist, La Lanne also considers himself a nutritionist, although why is a mystery. The only conceivable reason may be because he eats food. Unlike his predecessor, Bernarr MacFadden, La Lanne does recognize the importance of vitamins. But typical of the nutritional misguidance offered at his health salons is the "fact" that meat is a desirable food because it contains "vitamins A, B, C, D, and G." In reality, meat contains very little A and D, and the amount of C is almost negligible. As for "vitamin G," La Lanne is evidently the only contemporary "nutritionist" who ever heard of it. (Aside from those few inaccuracies, he is right in saying that meat, in moderation, is a desirable food.)

35

The emphasis on physical fitness was gradually accompanied, then exceeded, by an emphasis on superhealth. But the means to attain this "superhealth" was not only unscientific, but illogical. Use of dietary supplements consisting of vitamins, minerals, and other chemical compounds became common, sometimes to a dangerous extreme. Yet the very same people who shy away from "all those chemicals or additives" and proclaim, "I never eat processed food," do not understand that dietary supplements are the *most processed supplements to foods one can consume.*

OF ORGANIC CHICKENS AND HAPPY EGGS

The health-food industry and its gurus have fostered the fashion and fear in every conceivable way. Power of suggestion is amply put to work. Advertisements and placards in the stores greet us with, "Do you feel tired, run-down. . . ?" If you've just come from a hard day at the office or are escaping from a houseful of young children (even one child, if toddler age, may qualify as a houseful), the answer is probably, "Yes." (Or, "Yes!!") Another favorite is: "Do you have minor aches and pains you didn't used to have?" Well, if we think about it hard enough, most of us can conjure up a twinge or two we hadn't noticed yesterday. Some alfalfa meal will fix us right up, we're advised, along with a big bottle of vitamin E and some desiccated liver.

There are other plays on the emotions. We are warned of the inadequacies of unfertilized eggs, for instance. (Those are the kind normally found in most supermarkets today.) According to the health-food people, commercial chicken coops are a man-made disaster; only a happy hen that is free to pick and scratch and copulate at will can lay a healthy egg. To compound that bit of balderdash is the further contention that the eggs of free-roaming hens contain more lecithin, which allegedly "dissolves" the cholesterol therein and thus renders them "safe" to eat. Fact: Scientists know that fertilized eggs do not contain more lecithin; lecithin does not dissolve cholesterol; and, furthermore, the cholesterol in eggs is not harmful, assuming that your blood cholesterol level is not elevated and egg consumption is reasonable.

The medical profession has inadvertently done its part to contribute to nutrition quackery in a number of ways. First, because too few medical doctors educated a decade or more ago are trained in nutrition, some may perpetuate misinformation, such as advising high-dose supplements or cautioning patients to completely avoid white bread and refined sugar.

Second, all too often, medical counsel is shunned entirely. Many people have a basic mistrust and/or fear of doctors; they may have difficulty relating to physicians and tend to perceive them as cold and unsympathetic; and they often fail to realize that many diseases, particularly those with emotional roots, are difficult to diagnose and treat. A general lack of satisfaction may be coupled with a great deal of expense; perhaps an operation is indicated, or prolonged budget-draining medical treatment.

Irrationally, many people postpone a visit to the doctor because of dread that their worst suspicions will be realized. Or perhaps an incurable condition or fatal disease has already been diagnosed, and the patient is unwilling to accept the inevitable. Often, patients will dismiss medical help in favor of a "better" or cheaper method they have heard about elsewhere. A prime example is the countless sufferers who have succumbed to cancer because they chose useless Laetrile treatment instead of chemotherapy, radiation, or surgery that might have saved or prolonged their lives.

Whatever the reason, great numbers of individuals have a tendency to look to sources other than physicians for answers, and the health faddists stand ready to provide them. The phenomenon is hardly new. In the late sixteenth century, Francis Bacon wrote: "We see the weakness and credulity of men is such that they prefer the mountebank or witch before a learned physician."

HEALTH FOODS AND NATURAL NATURE

Of course, health-food-store proprietors and other misinformation leaders are not likely to relish the appellation of mountebanks or witches. In fact, many of them have even turned away from the term "health food," preferring instead such euphemisms as "nutritional centers," "natural-food shops," and "nature foods."

Regardless of the names given to these emporiums, questionable practices abound. One former health-food-store owner told a researcher from the American Council on Science and Health some disturbing stories about the practices in her former place of business. She said, "I feel [that health-food stores] are selling things just for the money, while they're perfectly well aware that iodine is not going to make the bald man's hair grow back, that vitamin E won't restore sexual potency. I am sure the owner knows these facts when he sells these items."

When asked if any medical problems had resulted from the use of herbs sold in her store, she told the interviewer, "Yes, snakeroot. Some people overdosed on it. In fact, one customer was hospitalized as a result of it."

Were there products that were labeled organic or natural, but really weren't? The former health-food-store owner said, "Yes, cucumbers and zucchini from [one company that sells organic/natural products] were waxed. Also, I frequently had local people sell me stuff they said was organic, but later I'd find it really wasn't, that they had sprayed it."

Why did she quit the health-food business? "I just didn't believe it anymore. It got to the point where I was almost hiding from my customers. I couldn't look them in the eye. After I stopped believing, I just couldn't sell it anymore."

If diet supplements and "wonder foods" are useless, why do so many people continue to buy them and insist they work? There are a number of reasons.

1) The products "cure" diseases that never existed in the first place. Hypoglycemia (low blood sugar) is a favorite here. Although in reality an extremely rare disease, health faddists and shop owners would have you believe it is overrunning the country.

2) Almost unanimously, scientific authorities agree that 80

percent of all disorders are self-limiting. In other words, they will cure themselves. The average cold will disappear in three to seven days if you take high doses of vitamin C. The average cold will also disappear in three to seven days if you do nothing at all. But as long as you are "doing something" for your cold, it is easy to assume that's what is "curing" it.

3) The Food and Drug Administration has reported that sick people are so eager to believe in "quick, easy, miraculous cure-alls" that it is next to impossible to convince them of a product's worthlessness or potential for harm. This eagerness enhances the "placebo effect" of many products; that is, a substance that is *supposed* to make one feel better often does, by the simple power of suggestion. (Remember Grandma's hot lemonade? And Jewish mothers for generations have known of the curative value of chicken soup.)*

4) The helplessness one feels when watching a loved one suffer is alleviated somewhat by providing almost any kind of remedy, whether it works or not.

5) Many people are vaguely anxious about other aspects of their life-styles, such as cigarette smoking, and feel they must compensate by doing "something extra" for their health.

6) People won't admit they've been swindled. In fact, they often go to great lengths to prove otherwise. After all, who wants to admit to having been a dummy, even temporarily?

Beware of Quackery

Up to now we've tried to avoid overuse of the word "quack," a term that originated during the Renaissance. At that time, mercury—or quicksilver—was a popular remedy for syphilis. Peddlers known as "quacksalvers" wandered about selling mercury ointments and claiming they would cure any illness. In due

* Actually, according to some recent scientific studies, chicken soup may indeed be helpful in treating colds, perhaps because it is a good source of fluids.

time the title was shortened to "quack." Cure-alls of today, of course, include almost everything *but* mercury.

Here are a few questions to ponder whenever you encounter magical claims for any kind of food or ingredient.

"Revolutionary" is a favorite description of many current theories and products. Consider: Has it been properly tested in several controlled studies? Does it conform with known scientific data? And is it really new?

"Used for generations to cure . . ." is a phrase often accompanied by a petulant complaint that physicians won't recommend it because they want your money. One health-food corporation expounds on the marvels of an herbal laxative that was "formulated fifty-five years ago." If it's so great, why has no one heard of it in all that time?

"It cured me of . . ." (or my Aunt Minnie or my neighbor's second cousin) immediately raises the question of who made the diagnosis. Many supposedly "cured" cases of cancer never exhibited any of the seven warning signs set up by the American Cancer Society—almost a sure sign that the disorder was *not* cancer. A self-cure for self-diagnosis often works—as long as the condition is something that is going to go away anyway.

"Organic" is a commonly misused term. All living matter is organic; what is frequently meant instead is "organically grown" (a topic we will discuss more fully in chapter 5). The expensive oranges you purchase in a health-food store may be labeled "organic," but that doesn't mean those in the supermarket are "inorganic." Similarly, a phrase like "pure organic iron" makes no sense: Iron is a mineral; therefore, in its "pure" state it can't possibly be organic.

But while quackery implies deliberate deceit, our concerns about misinformation are not limited to that particular aspect of the problem. Consider such ill-informed but popular misstatements as the following:

- Food additives in our diet are causing ill health.
- Reduction of cholesterol and saturated fats will, in itself,

protect the general population from heart disease and cancer.

- Sugar is a killer.
- The nutrition of American children is poor and made worse by the presence of something called "junk food."
- "Natural" foods or those grown by "organic" methods are better than other foods.
- Everyone needs vitamin supplements.
- The American public as a whole is poorly nourished.

Such allegations are at variance with scientific evidence and statistics on health in this country. The American public is being misled, victimized by a very expensive and health-threatening nutritional hoax.

The science of nutrition offers a vast amount of well-documented knowledge. Riding right alongside is a great deal of "maybe" knowledge—studies that indicate *possible* relationships, but which require far more research before becoming absolute fact.

Pitting what we do know against what has not yet become established fact can be a risky business. Major dietary changes advocated on the basis of premature evidence may well lead to conditions that are worse than those one is hoping to correct.

The following chapters take a look at the facts behind the popular nutritional claims. In them we attempt to separate fact from myth, and truth from conjecture. While you are reading, keep in mind that the material presented here is not simply the opinion of the authors. Rather, it represents the consensus of the vast majority of the nutritional, medical and public-health community.

CHAPTER 2

The Basic Premise of the Nutrition Hoax: Americans Are Undernourished

A FAVORITE ARGUMENT AMONG THOSE PRO-moting the nutrition hoax is that almost every person in the United States is suffering from borderline nutrition deficiency. This appeal to fear is not only untrue, it ignores the fact that the major forms of "poor" nourishment in this country have to do with overeating (and resulting obesity) by a high percentage of almost every segment of the population, and with undernutrition only in certain poverty-stricken areas.

Healthy People, the Surgeon General's *Report on Health Promotion and Disease Prevention,* assured us in 1979 that "less than one percent of the American people can be considered under-nourished in the traditional sense." That conclusion was based on comprehensive national data obtained from the first Health and Nutrition Examination Survey (HANES) conducted by the National Center for Health Statistics. Their findings agreed with the trends indicated by numerous other nutrition studies during the past several years. Yet everyone from politicians to vitamin packagers continues to disregard numerical fact, each clinging devotedly to his own baseless theory.

We list here a few of the unfounded charges being hurled by would-be health pushers. They represent only pure speculation and opinion:

- Carlton Fredericks, in *Look Younger, Feel Healthier,* tells us that "borderline deficiency is the most vicious type of malnutrition." He ballyhoos the lavish use of his favorite super-supplements along with the "benefits we can achieve by ignoring the dictates of the Nutritional Establishment" (capital letters his).
- Dr. Michael F. Jacobson in *Eater's Digest* points an accusatory finger at the capitalistic world of business: "It is unlikely that, behind the closed boardroom doors of this nation's food and chemical companies, the managers are grappling with the problem of how to solve once and for all America's problems of hunger and malnutrition. More likely they are calculating how they can increase sales and asking how food additives can help."
- In *The Complete Junk Food Book,* Michael S. Lasky admonishes: "The excessive consumption of junk food is, if not killing us slowly, gradually making us malnourished and unhealthy."
- In *Megavitamins: A New Key to Health,* Lynn Lilliston quotes the blusterings of Senator William Proxmire ("a physical-fitness buff") about the removal of wheat germ from white bread: "As a result, the American people probably eat the poorest, least nutritious white bread of any modern, industrialized, civilized nation." Wheat germ is removed in the process of making flour, from which white bread is made the world over. In the United States, federal enrichment laws require that some of the nutrients lost in this processing be put back into the white bread.
- The same book also quotes Dr. Abram Hoffer, one of two

43

psychiatrists who pioneered megavitamin therapy as a "cure" for schizophrenia: "Senility is due to chronic malnutrition—it is a vitamin-dependent condition which comes from many years of mild or moderate chronic vitamin deficiency." There is no scientific evidence to support this claim for megavitamins, or that senility is caused by lack of vitamins.

- In *Pure and Simple,* Marian Burros, former food editor of the *Washington Post* and now a food writer at the *New York Times,* has us somewhat confused by stating, "Some additives . . . replace the expensive valuable nutrients with cheap ones to increase profitability." (Our problem: How does one distinguish between a cheap nutrient and an expensive one; and what do the industrialists do with those "expensive valuable nutrients" after removing them from food? It sounds as though they carry them to the bank.)

- Dr. Lendon Smith, in *Feed Your Kids Right,* chides us: "We could all be healthier than we are, and the failure to achieve an elevated plateau is directly proportional to the degree and significance of our various nutritional deficiencies."

- In *The Great Nutrition Robbery,* Beatrice Trum Hunter berates the manufacturers of synthetic foods: "Although great attention is given to approximating appearance, taste, texture, and other characteristics of real foods, the subject of nutritional value is ignored." Two examples she cites are imitation cheeses formulated from "banana peels, ground-up buttons, and umbrella handles"; and experimental cookies in which some of the flour has been replaced by ground-up chicken feathers. Her objection to the latter is that the protein in feathers is incomplete, and therefore that ingredient is inferior. (It's all a matter of preference, of course, but we do not personally advocate the use of either chicken feathers or ground buttons as an important part of the diet. Esthetically, something seems to be missing.)

Antiproof: The Actual Statistics

In contrast, let's take a look at what has *really* been happening on the national nutrition scene.

In the 1930s, it was estimated that approximately one-third of all American families were poorly fed. As the Great Depression passed into the history books, increasingly nutritious meals began to appear on American dining tables. Added to this was a big push toward nutrition education during World War II (a push that today needs to be expanded), as well as the evolution of enrichment policies during those years. Also, through advanced technology in food processing and preservation, a larger variety of food became available to the public at reasonable cost.

"Enrichment" or "fortification"—the process of replacing major nutrients which were lost during food processing, up to specific legal standards—was of particular importance as applied to breads and cereals. Those foods comprised a substantial portion of the American diet at that time. In the enrichment program, iron and B vitamins—niacin, riboflavin, and thiamine—were (and still are) added to white flour up to the levels present in whole wheat flour. Once this was done, people had little difficulty in fulfilling their daily requirements for these nutrients, whether their breads and cereals consisted of whole grain products or otherwise. The argument is frequently voiced that white bread, even though enriched, is still inferior to whole grain bread because the trace nutrients have not been replaced. While that statement is true, it does not take into account that the missing trace nutrients are easily available in other foods that we eat as part of a balanced diet. If one were to limit his dietary intake to bread and cereal (white or brown, and with or without sugar), he would be missing out on a lot more than just trace nutrients.

By 1955, comprehensive government studies indicated that only about one family in ten consumed a diet that was nutritionally poor. The studies further revealed that nutritional inadequacy was due more to lack of knowledge than to poverty. But nutritionally educated or not, that still left 10 percent of the population about which to be concerned.

The establishment of school-lunch programs, the advent of food stamps, and the WIC (Women, Infants and Children) program, projects sponsored by state and local governments, as well as the efforts of various community-service groups have all contributed enormously toward continually improved diets for everyone. In addition, countless technological advancements have made it possible for thousands of new items to appear on grocers' shelves and, ultimately, on our tables. In almost every section of the country, new processing techniques and transportation facilities offer easily accessible ingredients for a varied, balanced diet, regardless of season.

How consumer advocate Dr. Michael F. Jacobson is able to complain, in a book published in 1972, that "a smaller fraction of Americans received adequate amounts of nutrients in 1965 than in 1955" is something of an enigma. As we have already mentioned, the most recent, thoroughly documented figures available bear out the trends toward improved nutrition that began almost half a century ago. We refer, of course, to the HANES (Health and Nutrition Examination Survey) study, a project encompassing nearly 21,000 persons, aged 1–74, during the years 1971–74. *Vital and Health Statistics,* published by HEW, describes the survey as "the first program to collect measures of nutritional status from a scientifically designed sample representative of the U.S. civilian noninstitutionalized population in a broad range of ages."

The tables on the following pages reveal that the overwhelming majority of Americans are more than meeting Recommended Dietary Allowances (RDA) for protein, calcium, thiamine, riboflavin, and vitamins A and C. If people meet these allowances by eating foods, and not by taking supplements, the chances are very good they will receive more than adequate amounts of all other nutrients. These figures are percentages; therefore, any number over 100 is in excess of the recommended allowance. Of particular interest is the similarity of the figures for groups above and below poverty level.

Another important observation is the level of excess consumption shown for various nutrients. For example, many Americans are consuming an average of twice the RDA for protein. In addition, the RDA for protein was lowered from 65 g/day to 56 g/day for an average adult male in 1974.

THE EXCEPTION

But while this major study indicates that less than 1 percent of the citizenry is undernourished, there is one notable exception, quite obvious from the tables.

That exception is the iron level in the diets of women during the childbearing years (due to the loss of blood during menstruation), as well as in children during their preschool years. Factors contributing to iron deficiency in early life include: low stores at birth, especially in prematures; low iron content of milk and high requirement for rapid growth. Another leading component in iron deficiency is the fact that only a small percentage of the dietary iron consumed is actually absorbed by the human body. Despite the statistics, however, iron seems to have fallen from the popularity it enjoyed for so many years. We can only assume that is because this very basically necessary mineral lacks much of the glamour and many of the deceptive promises attributed to other nutrients (with which almost every diet is already supplied in abundance).

Iron is necessary for many metabolic reactions, particularly for the production of hemoglobin. Hemoglobin is what determines the oxygen-carrying potential of our red blood cells. If you are a woman below the age of fifty or so, and frequently feel fatigued and listless, it is possible that your problem is caused by a deficiency of plain old-fashioned iron. But check with your doctor! These symptoms can have many causes, and most have nothing to do with diet. Health-food pushers would have you believe that your lethargy must be of dietary origin and would cite almost everything else as a possible cause (including the additives in

Table 1. Mean, Protein, Calcium, and Iron Intakes of Persons Aged 1–74 Years as a Percent of Standard for Income Levels, by Sex and Age: United States, 1971–74

Sex and age	Protein			Calcium			Iron		
	All income	Below poverty level[1]	Above poverty level[1]	All income	Below poverty level[1]	Above poverty level[1]	All income	Below poverty level[1]	Above poverty level[1]
	Percent of standard								
Male									
1 year	235	240	235	207	203	208	50	47	51
2–3 years	230	240	226	194	193	193	55	54	55
4–5 years	231	220	233	223	188	231	94	90	95
6–7 years	265	275	264	243	214	258	112	114	111
8–9 years	212	216	211	258	226	267	113	113	112
10–11 years	193	166	199	185	155	190	127	114	129
12–14 years	158	145	161	198	158	205	96	99	97
15–17 years	154	133	157	229	201	232	91	74	93
18–19 years	156	142	156	227	181	234	92	88	92
20–24 years	143	125	146	279	242	281	165	143	168
25–34 years	142	139	142	262	194	267	167	172	167
35–44 years	134	142	134	229	278	226	159	164	159
45–54 years	125	114	126	210	186	212	146	126	147
55–64 years	113	91	117	194	193	196	137	111	141
65 years and over	99	91	102	179	152	184	121	113	123

Female

1 year	240	234	242	202	196	204	48	37	51
2–3 years	221	221	221	190	170	195	48	48	48
4–5 years	217	232	214	199	192	201	84	88	83
6–7 years	224	223	225	222	210	226	96	89	98
8–9 years	179	194	177	223	208	228	97	106	96
10–11 years	171	176	170	169	129	178	58	64	57
12–14 years	120	118	120	148	131	152	58	61	57
15–17 years	99	88	101	131	106	137	53	46	54
18–19 years	114	107	117	130	116	137	56	53	57
20–24 years	104	94	105	111	100	113	56	53	56
25–34 years	105	98	106	107	91	109	57	54	58
35–44 years	103	94	103	100	88	101	58	51	58
45–54 years	108	97	107	99	93	99	59	52	59
55–64 years	98	80	99	96	90	97	97	81	98
65 years and over	90	84	92	95	88	97	92	80	96

[1] Excludes persons with unknown income.

Source: "Caloric and Selected Nutrient Values for Persons 1–74 Years of Age: First Health and Nutrition Examination Survey, United States, 1971–1974." Vital and Health Statistics, DHEW Publication No. (PHS) 79-1657. U.S. Department of Health, Education and Welfare; Public Health Service; Office of Health Research, Statistics, and Technology; National Center for Health Statistics; Hyattsville (Md.), June 1979.

Table 2. Mean Vitamin A, Vitamin C, Thiamine, and Riboflavin Intakes of Persons Aged 1–74 Years as a Percent of Standard for Income Levels, by Sex and Age: United States, 1971–74

Sex and age	Vitamin A			Vitamin C			Thiamine			Riboflavin		
	All income	Below poverty level[1]	Above poverty level[1]	All income	Below poverty level[1]	Above poverty level[1]	All income	Below poverty level[1]	Above poverty level[1]	All income	Below poverty level[1]	Above poverty level[1]
	Percent of standard											
Male												
1 year	189	226	182	175	136	186	175	165	178	242	245	240
2–3 years	180	199	176	209	186	215	173	178	170	205	205	204
4–5 years	189	197	189	214	181	223	170	175	168	198	182	202
6–7 years	175	184	171	205	173	217	163	165	163	195	178	202
8–9 years	186	167	191	196	176	201	150	147	152	195	175	200
10–11 years	207	157	210	223	125	233	165	170	163	191	181	193
12–14 years	157	165	154	195	168	205	158	170	150	184	185	184
15–17 years	166	125	172	195	170	199	152	150	152	173	171	173
18–19 years	161	104	166	212	173	216	147	153	145	165	154	167
20–24 years	152	139	150	180	153	186	150	157	147	160	167	156
25–34 years	153	146	151	150	103	152	153	165	160	160	158	158
35–44 years	153	175	149	138	129	139	147	160	147	160	171	158
45–54 years	148	142	149	140	115	143	155	157	157	163	160	163
55–64 years	163	133	166	160	114	165	165	163	166	171	183	171
65 years and over	157	113	167	147	107	156	172	170	172	178	167	180

Female

1 year	176	155	182	160	117	170	193	165	196	258	253	258
2–3 years	174	163	175	182	162	186	173	175	170	218	216	218
4–5 years	178	181	176	198	179	203	165	170	165	200	191	202
6–7 years	146	159	143	199	177	206	163	158	165	193	187	195
8–9 years	158	210	150	210	254	202	165	175	163	193	185	185
10–11 years	161	166	162	208	192	213	158	170	152	187	165	191
12–14 years	124	128	123	174	154	177	160	165	160	181	171	184
15–17 years	102	89	108	143	143	146	158	140	163	175	153	181
18–19 years	114	109	118	186	176	187	157	160	157	163	145	170
20–24 years	106	108	106	153	148	154	165	163	163	163	156	165
25–34 years	122	105	125	138	113	140	163	163	163	171	158	173
35–44 years	120	98	122	145	116	149	163	160	165	167	163	167
45–54 years	152	218	149	150	107	153	170	163	170	178	213	176
55–64 years	177	142	179	178	122	183	180	170	180	193	178	194
65 years and over	148	126	157	164	130	174	185	182	185	193	191	194

[1] Excludes persons with unknown income.
Source: Ibid.

processed foods), but for some unexplainable reason they place very little emphasis on iron. Of course, iron is offered in the form of desiccated liver, but that probably doesn't appeal to too many people other than hard-core enthusiasts. Sometimes it is advertised as an ingredient in various other concoctions, such as Geritol, but those remedies are often shunned because they have the ring of "patent medicine." The cost of iron from such tonics is far greater than the cost of iron from simple iron pills of ferrous sulfate.

Another factor contributing to iron deficiency is decreased consumption of bread (made with enriched flour) in recent years, especially among women. Somewhere along the line, bread was mistakenly dubbed "fattening," and weight watchers began to avoid it. An average slice of bread contains only seventy calories. It makes little sense to pass up the bread in favor of an extra serving of meat that has far more calories, though it should be mentioned that meat is the best source of readily absorbable iron.

We find it curious that although females between the ages of ten and fifty-four years (a sizable portion of the population) barely exceed *50 percent* of their recommended allowance of iron, so little attention is paid to this nutrient by food faddists. Yet vitamin C, on the other hand, is hawked continually, even though all age groups average about one and a half to two times their recommended allowance of this nutrient, indicating that most of us consume ample amounts of vitamin C. It should also be mentioned that vitamin C favors the absorption of iron. This important benefit is seldom mentioned by those advising the increased consumption of vitamin C.

If you are suffering from iron-deficiency anemia, your physician will probably recommend iron supplements for a time. But it is important that you also get into the habit of including enough iron-rich foods in your daily diet.

ANYTHING ELSE?

There are two additional exceptions not apparent from the tables but that we feel require a brief mention. One is that in most parts of the country there is insufficient fluoride in the food and water supply to reduce tooth decay unless this nutrient is added to community drinking water. Hundreds, maybe even thousands, of reputable studies have shown repeatedly that if the fluoride content of water is adjusted to 1 ppm (part per million), it will substantially decrease the incidence of dental caries (by 60–70 percent in those who have had access to fluoridated water from birth). Yet, nationwide, local crusaders have fought tooth and nail against this simple public-health measure. And, of course, health-food promoters never mention it. The reason is obvious enough: There is no money to be made from fluoride in the drinking water; they would much prefer to sell you bone meal or dolomite as a tooth-decay preventative. And unknowing people continue to buy these products, even though scientists know there is no factual basis for the claims made for either one.

Second, women on the Pill, or anyone on any kind of prolonged medication, need to be especially cautious about consuming a balanced diet. Some drugs tend to interfere with normal nutrient metabolism. In the case of the oral contraceptive pill, if this occurs at all, it is only to a small degree and does not require the addition of any kind of supplement *so long as* the daily diet is well balanced. Other drugs may have more significant effects. If you are taking any type of long-term medication that may interfere with normal absorption or metabolism of a vitamin or mineral, your physician is more than likely to be aware of that effect and will prescribe accordingly.

DEFICIENCY DISEASE

Purveyors of commercial diet supplements have historically made the most of nutrition surveys that indicate *any* kind of deficiency (with the odd exception of iron, mentioned above). Most popular are claims that Americans are tending to develop deficiencies of every sort of trace nutrient—claims that can't always be readily disproven, since trace nutrients are rarely included in large national studies. But the reasons they are not should be fairly obvious: a) If one is consuming sufficient amounts of foods providing the major nutrients, it is most likely that he is also consuming sufficient amounts of the minor ones; b) deficiencies of nutrients included in tables 1 and 2 are so rare (except for iron), that specific widespread testing is not feasible.

For instance, it is virtually impossible in the modern world for an adult to consume a diet deficient in vitamin E. In fact, when the early researchers who discovered that vitamin attempted to learn what would happen to laboratory animals deprived of it, they found their most difficult task was planning a diet that would create a vitamin E deficiency. As another example, our main source of vitamin K is the bacteria normally present in our intestines (they make it, and we absorb it). Normal adults, therefore, have an adequate supply of vitamin K without ingesting any at all.

The classic diseases of vitamin deficiency, such as beriberi, scurvy, and rickets, are rarities in the United States today. Generally speaking, a true deficiency of any nutrient other than iron and fluoride is not easy to produce in our society. The shortage must necessarily be extreme, and it must persist over a considerable period of time.

Man is able to maintain good health with a rather wide range of nutrient intake, and short-term deficits are easily restored. In *Food and Your Well-Being,* Dr. Theodore P. Labuza of the University of Minnesota points out that the Recommended Dietary Allowance for any nutrient "is a standard that does not have to be met exactly." What is of concern from a health standpoint is when people fall below 50 to 60 percent of the RDA, and for a period of time. Furthermore, the Food and Nutrition Board, which sets the RDA, states that "RDA [except for energy] are estimated to *exceed* the requirements of most individuals, and thereby ensure that the needs of nearly all are met."

Deficiency diseases *do* exist, of course, but very rarely, and they require medical testing and diagnosis in order to be identified. An insufficiency of a single vitamin or mineral is almost impossible for a layman to discern, although many health-food sellers are quick to hand out diagnoses right and left. Furthermore, if because of an improper diet a person is deficient in one nutrient, he is probably deficient in several. (The solution: a balanced diet based on the Basic Four Food Groups, not a host of supplements.)

A nutritional deficiency that does not result from improper eating habits usually indicates a special health problem whereby the vitamin or mineral is consumed in sufficient amounts but is not metabolized properly. A classic case is pernicious anemia, which results from a defect in the body's ability to absorb vitamin B_{12} from the gastrointestinal tract and get it into the rest of the body, where it is needed. When the hucksters advise oral supplements of vitamin B_{12} to prevent or treat this disease, they are doling out nonsense. Extra B_{12} taken orally will not prevent or cure pernicious anemia. Oral supplements are not used in its treatment quite simply because the digestive tract is where the problem is. Instead, injected vitamin B_{12} must be used to bypass the gastrointestinal system. And you can't buy injectable vitamins at your local health-food store.

A vitamin B_{12} deficiency can also result from a dietary insufficiency, although such cases are rare. The condition is found primarily in total vegetarians (vegans) because the only dietary sources of B_{12} are foods of animal origin.

PLANT MALNUTRITION?

Another favorite quack argument is that soil depletion and artificial fertilizers are causing malnutrition. The fertilizer fallacy will be discussed more fully in chapter 5. Here we will merely note that if needed nutrients are missing from the soil, a plant simply will not grow properly. Otherwise, the nutritional levels of edible plant portions (except for some minerals) are very little affected by how they have been grown—and certainly not by the type of fertilizer used.

We're Not Immortal

Those who speak so fondly of the "good old days" obviously didn't live in them. Death is always a tragedy. It cannot be construed as either more or less tragic today than it was generations ago. The difference is that for the average person of the 1980s, the inevitable is likely to occur at a much later age than it did a century ago.

Infectious diseases have largely been conquered. Development of antibiotics, immunization programs, improved sanitation, and a heightened knowledge of both nutrition and general health practices have all contributed to the conquest. In 1900, the leading cause of death in the United States was tuberculosis—194.4 persons out of every 100,000 (that's almost 1 in 500). By 1976, that 194.4 figure had been reduced to 1.5. Pneumonia, the second leading cause of death at the turn of the century, has enjoyed a decline that is only slightly less striking. And, except in a few rare and isolated cases, diseases like diphtheria, whooping cough, measles, and polio are no longer common or fatal in the United States.

Obviously, if Americans are less likely to die from infectious diseases, then they are *more* likely to die from noninfectious diseases, such as heart disease, and at a later age. If a loved one dies of cancer, there is little consolation in knowing that at an earlier period in our history he or she would probably have died twenty years sooner from pneumonia or TB. Nevertheless, that is the picture we have before us today.

''KILLER DISEASES''
Beyond the bounds of logic is the popular premise that America is now in the midst of an "epidemic" of noninfectious "killer diseases" (to borrow two of former Senator George McGovern's terms). The favorite corollary is that most of these "killers" are allegedly related to faulty nutrition:

- *Dietary Goals for the United States,* prepared in 1977 by the Senate Select Committee on Nutrition and Human Needs (the so-called "McGovern Committee"), suggested that diet has been linked with "six of the ten leading causes of death: heart disease, cancer, cerebrovascular disease (stroke), diabetes, arteriosclerosis, and cirrhosis of the liver." In the foreword, Senator McGovern begins: "The purpose of this report is to point out that the eating patterns of this century represent as critical a public health concern as any now before us."

Ever since the preliminary data for *Dietary Goals* were released, healthmongers have seized and run off with the study's nationally criticized tenets. We mention here only two brief examples, but they are typical of numerous others echoing the same ill-advised battle cry:

- In a recent interview, Joan Dye Gussow, chairperson of the Program of Nutrition Education at Teachers College, Columbia University (completely separate from the Department of Nutrition, School of Public Health, Columbia University) told *FDA Consumer:* "Something has been undercutting what should be steady progress toward health. And I don't think you can escape the conclusion that improper diet is a major contributing factor. . . . The increasing rates of cancer, heart disease, and diabetes are all suggestive of a complex of problems that seem to be related to diet factors."
- Michael S. Lasky, in *The Complete Junk Food Book,* asserts, "Various authorities have informed us many times that [junk food] contributes to tooth rot and causes diabetes, heart ailments, and cancer."

The American population is aging significantly. Life expectancy has increased by twenty years since 1900, with the result that a growing proportion of citizens now belong to that group known as the elderly. In 1900, only 4 percent of Americans were over sixty-five years of age; by 1975, that figure had risen to 10 percent, and all indications are that the percentage will continue to rise. Dr. Paola Timiras, a gerontologist, recently predicted that by 1985 the American population seventy years and over will rise by 11 percent for men and 14 percent for women.

As one passes middle age, the risk of falling victim to one of the degenerative diseases—heart disease, cancer, adult-onset diabetes, arthritis, or obesity, for example—increases. As more and more people live beyond middle age, the incidence of degenerative-type diseases increases proportionately. Until medical science advances far beyond its present state, humans will necessarily continue to die from *something*. The greatly increased death rates from cardiovascular diseases and from cancer (but from the latter only when the rates are not adjusted for age) can be readily explained by three factors: a) Years ago great numbers of people did not live long enough to develop degenerative diseases; b) control of infectious diseases has resulted in proportionately more deaths caused by the noninfectious or degenerative diseases; and c) inferior diagnostic methods of past years did not always determine the exact cause of death.

Progress is being made. Although still the number-one cause of death in the United States, the heart-disease death rate has begun to decline—a 30 percent decrease since 1950. This would be good news indeed were it not for a rise in lung-cancer deaths. But are these noninfectious diseases *diet*-related? Let's consider a few facts:

1) The only type of cancer death that has appreciably increased has been lung cancer—and that is directly attributable to cigarette smoking, not diet.
2) Deaths from stomach cancer have actually shown a steady decline during the past fifty years.
3) In 1900, gastrointestinal disturbances like diarrhea and enteritis took the lives of 140 out of every 100,000 persons. By 1976, the figure was reduced to fewer than one person in every 100,000.
4) During the years since 1900, when life expectancy was

being lengthened by twenty years, consumption of refined foods gradually increased at the same time.

Where is the epidemic?

IS DIET INVOLVED AT ALL?

We do not presume to say that degenerative-type diseases are *never* diet-related. Indications are that some forms of some diseases in some individuals may very well be affected by certain dietary excesses. But with few exceptions (for instance, the association between salt and the 20 percent of the population that develops hypertension), scientists just don't know very much yet about the role of diet in the etiology of these degenerative-type diseases. We do know that good nutrition is an underlying key to good health and that obesity is a hazard, but precise relationships are generally still very "iffy" at this point. Conversely, a number of other factors have been definitely established as casually related to disorders like cancer and heart disease. We will take a closer look at those risk factors in chapters 4 and 6.

In other words, what we are saying is that popping vitamin pills every few hours, or avoiding white bread and refined sugar, is not going to either cure or prevent degenerative disease. Certain dietary modifications may be in order, but extremes are not. What too many people fail to realize is that there are other lifestyle factors on which to focus their attention that *will* reduce their risks. You may be disappointed, but there simply are no wonder supplements or magic potions.

We're Not Undernourished, But We're Trying

For the most part, our nation is not undernourished right now. But increasingly eccentric eating habits, fad diets, and the spread of misinformation may be *creating* faulty nutrition.

Evidently, America loves paradox. It almost seems unfair that certain breads and cereals—the first items to be enriched and fortified in a government effort to improve nutrition—are now under the greatest attack as inferior foods. Many supermarkets, joining the "natural" march, are moving such items as whole wheat flour and wheat germ to newly created "health-food" sections. And, of course, a "rise in status" calls for a rise in price. So what is happening is that these perfectly nutritious foods are actually *less* available to the low-income shopper. Either she (or he) guiltily buys instead what she fears is an inferior product, or she pays the higher prices and does without other needed food items.

The White House Conference on Food, Nutrition and Health of just over a decade ago attributed malnutrition not so much to an overall shortage of available nutrients as to a lack of consumer knowledge of nutrition and "actual misinformation disseminated in advertising and other communications media." And Dr. George Briggs, of the University of California at Berkeley, told a congressional hearing that "poor nutrition [is mostly] caused by misinformation."

The American Medical Association House of Delegates in the mid 1970s adopted the following summary statement on the matter: "Most people have little genuine knowledge about the science of nutrition; what they call 'nutrition' is not likely to be founded in science at all. The public is continually distracted by announcements of hazards associated with foods, food additives, or various dietary practices. Many warnings are unfounded or premature, but the fears thus engendered adversely influence attitudes about foods. The public is also misled by extravagant claims of health benefits derived from the use of certain foods or nutrient supplements."

In an honest effort to achieve better health, millions of consumers are believing and following nutrition misinformation—and it extends from infancy through old age.

FEEDING THE BABY

Both home- and commercially prepared baby foods are fine for most babies. But no matter which type of food is used, knowledge of nutrient content of foods and of babies' nutritional needs are basic for proper food selection and preparation.

Parents may be aware that babies prefer bland food; what they often don't realize is just how very flat that blandness can be. As a result, parents often unnecessarily add salt or sugar to baby foods they prepare themselves, seasoning them to their tastes, not the babies' tastes! Then, too, there is the problem of proper storage of leftovers. Since babies are more sensitive to contamination than adults, greater care must be exercised to preserve the sanitary condition of their foods. Either way—with properly home-prepared or commercial foods—reasonable precautions will ensure that your baby's health is not impaired.

THE YEARS AFTER

The misinformation nutrition hoax doesn't wane after babyhood; it picks up speed:

• An older child is frequently fed granola these days in place of more traditional cereals. Granola, the healthmongers and advertisers tell us, is supposed to be all natural and therefore better for us and our children than most other varieties full of additives. But these unfounded claims merely serve to sell the product. Granolas, incidentally, have appreciably more calories than cereals, and that doesn't help the "obesity problem." In addition, a number of the more traditional cereals are enriched with a number of essential vitamins and minerals, which granola does not supply.

• Universities throughout the country have been forced in one way or another to open "health-food" cafeterias. Their offerings are adequate, of course, if they are used as part of a balanced diet, rather than as an encouragement toward fad diets. But these are a reflection of the extent to which food faddism has influenced the younger generation.

• A pregnant woman, in attempting to follow an ill-advised dietary-supplement regimen, may cause untold damage to her unborn baby. For example, megadoses of vitamin C during pregnancy may cause an infant to be born vitamin C-dependent. This means that such an infant would develop scurvy when supplied with the amount of vitamin C customarily recommended for infants.

• Edwin Bayrd points out in *The Thin Game:* "Men and women over the age of sixty-five need less of certain vitamins such as thiamine than do people under twenty-five, yet the elderly are the principal buyers of multivitamin tablets."

• Our nation's farming methods have been much maligned in recent years. But if modern agricultural technology were to be discarded in favor of organic farming, the cost of ordinary food would transform it to a luxury for most families. And worldwide, problems of hunger, malnutrition, and famine would be multiplied.

We have made a great deal of progress toward establishing America as the best-nourished country in the world. It would be folly indeed to allow this achievement to diminish because of unwarranted dietary changes.

The health huckster wailing on his soapbox about the miseries of American food is, as usual, displaying a patent disregard of the facts.

TOO MUCH FOOD?

There does exist in the United States today a far greater danger than undernutrition—it is the danger of a disproportionate amount of eating in relation to physical activity. That problem is a very real one. In fact, it is the subject of our next chapter.

CHAPTER 3

Obesity in America: Our Number-one Nutrition Problem

THERE IS ONE TOPIC ABOUT WHICH NUTRI-tion scientists are in almost unanimous agreement: The greatest nutritional problem in the United States today is obesity.

The percentages vary. Some estimates indicate that 30 percent of all American adults exceed their Desirable Weight—that's 70 to 80 million people. The Department of Health and Human Services statistics show that the average man is eighteen pounds and the average woman twenty-one pounds over his or her Desirable Weight. The nation's youth are not immune either: Recent studies by the President's Council on Physical Fitness and Sports indicate that one in three young Americans is also in this category. But in the absence of high blood pressure, high blood lipids, or diabetes, obesity becomes medically significant only at about 20 percent above the Desirable Weight. It is at this point that death rates exceed normal levels.

A Weighty Matter

There are a couple of reasons why estimates of the actual number of people who weigh too much are hard to evaluate. One is that the terms "overweight" and "obese" are often erroneously used interchangeably. *Overweight* indicates any poundage in excess of one's Desirable Weight. You are considered medically *obese* if you are more than 20 percent above Desirable Weight. Of those 70 to 80 million overweight Americans mentioned above, about 40 million are obese. About two-thirds of those are past the age of forty, and more than three-quarters of them are women. The recent Surgeon General's report, *Healthy People,* reveals that obesity is a slightly greater problem among women below poverty level than among those who are above poverty level. This may be because thin is considered chic, and higher socioeconomic circles place more emphasis on this. Therefore, wealthier women may be more conscious of keeping their weight down. For men the figures are reversed: More than two and a half times as many men above poverty level are obese compared to those who are below—a holdover, perhaps, from the days when a fat belly indicated prosperity.

Another reason for the discrepancy in the number of overweight may have to do with the time of year the figures were compiled. Most of us are only too well aware that the winter holidays are bad news for weight watchers. But when warm weather approaches, it strikes the signal for a mass reducing effort as sun worshipers prepare to wriggle into last year's swimwear.

HOW DID SO MANY PEOPLE GET SO FAT?

A life-style considered sedentary at the turn of the century would be regarded today as very active. People burned up a lot of calories in those days, and, except for those too poor to buy enough food, they necessarily consumed large amounts in order to maintain their energy balance. But the past eighty years have brought us labor-saving devices in great variety. People no longer burn anywhere near as many calories—but they've kept right on eating them. And anyone who eats more than his body expends in energy is going to gain weight. The simple weight-stabilizing equation of *calories in* = *calories out* tips out of balance.

When the scale pointer skidded too far toward the upper limits a few decades ago, it was a fairly simple matter just to eat a little less until it receded again. Most people were active enough that they could lose weight without making major concessions at mealtime. But as physical exercise decreased, dieting difficulties increased. Today's reducing diets must be restricted to about 1,200–1,500 calories for most overweight people, and that doesn't leave much margin for error if all of the recommended dietary allowances of nutrients are to be fitted in. The rise in alcoholic-beverage consumption hasn't helped much either, since alcohol contributes calories, but not many additional nutrients, to the diet. Anyone who could invent a two-calorie cocktail would become an instant millionaire.

Calories are sneaky. Edwin Bayrd, author of *The Thin Game*, has calculated that a mere ten minutes of exercise dropped from the daily schedule will result in a weight gain of four pounds a year. A single slice of chocolate layer cake (or its equivalent) eaten every day in excess of one's usual calorie requirement can lead to a weight gain of up to forty pounds in a year.

Great numbers of those overweight millions do try to lose their excess baggage. In fact, Bayrd estimates that half of all Americans spend one-quarter of their adult life dieting, encompassing about fifteen major diets each between the ages of twenty and fifty. That ought to tell you something right there. If the diets really worked, there would be no need to start a new one every few months.

The big problem is that far too many people fall for the gimmicky fad diets, the ones that promise you'll lose twenty pounds or so the first month, usually by some "revolutionary" new method that in actual fact is not the least bit revolutionary. You really may lose twenty pounds in a month. But then what happens? You go off the diet, return to your former eating habits, and those lost pounds reappear like magic. The faster you've lost it, the faster you'll gain it back. And that is precisely why 90 to 95 percent of all reducing diets ultimately fail. *The dieter retains the same bad habits—too many calories (food and drink) and too little exercise—that allowed those extra pounds to accumulate in the first place.* He has not learned to control weight by a proper balance of food and physical activity; he has simply suffered for a few weeks. But of more importance to health than feelings of failure, the rapid regain of weight is bad for the cardiovascular system. Rapid weight gain results in higher levels of blood cholesterol and an acceleration of the rate of cholesterol being deposited in the blood vessels, leading to accelerated promotion of arterial plaques—not good!

Any diet that deviates radically from sound nutrition principles is suspect and unsafe. Far too often, legitimate research results are misinterpreted and thus become the basis for a fad diet. Some advocate no fat, or no carbohydrates, or even no solid food at all. Others insist that a particular food must be eaten at every meal, or every day, or never. Many such diets are health hazards. All of them are useless. You cannot achieve permanent weight control until you learn how to handle, in moderation, all of the foods that make up a normal balanced diet. That doesn't mean you can't *ever* eat any of that chocolate layer cake, but it does mean you ought not to do it very often, unless you start moving around a lot more and eating *smaller portions.*

"BUT I'VE ALWAYS BEEN FAT— I'M USED TO IT"

One-third of all overweight adults were overweight as children. A child with one obese parent is 40 percent more likely to grow into an obese adult. If both parents are obese, the chances of the child becoming obese rise to 80 percent. Thus, the weight problem perpetuates itself.

Exactly what role heredity plays in obesity is still open to speculation. Studies indicate that overfed babies and young adolescents form more fat cells than others, a condition that appears to linger throughout one's lifetime and may explain why some adults gain weight more readily than others with the same general life-style and eating patterns. The underlying theory is that in early life the adipose (fat) tissue grows by increasing the number and/or the size of fat cells, while later in life the tissue grows only by increasing cell size.

Statistics tell us that girl babies generally have less body weight but higher fat content than boy babies, a factor that might influence the fact that three times as many women as men have a weight problem in adulthood. But simply being female is not a valid excuse for being fat. There is no doubt that life-style factors are the major contributors to the state of one's weight. The relationship between obese parent and obese children is not so much a matter of genetics as it is a tendency to learn basic habits in the family setting. If a parent overeats, a child is likely to do the same. Similarly, parents who are not very active tend to be less eager about encouraging physical activity in their offspring. Weight control, as with all other aspects of child rearing, requires that Mom and Pop begin by setting good examples.

The stereotype of the "jolly fat person" is largely a myth. Fat people may *look* comical, but their jovial ho-ho-ho's are all too often a compensatory measure, a combination apology and survival kit. They may have become accustomed to their corpulence, but they rarely become completely accustomed to their diminished attractiveness and the difficulty of finding fashionable clothing (a problem which still exists, although the clothing industry has recently made considerable progress in this area). No matter how cheerful the outward appearance, the facts are not to be laughed at. An obese person is like an accident waiting to happen—at increased risk of almost all fatal diseases.

There are other considerations as well. Many employers are consciously or subconsciously reluctant to hire the overweight. This is a form of discrimination, of course, but in some cases the employers may have legitimate reasons for preferring employees of normal weight. For instance, in some positions an unattractive appearance is a real disadvantage. Also, employers may be aware that obesity can be a sign of underlying physical or psychological conditions that could interfere with job performance. Discrimination against fat people isn't limited to job opportunities, either. Recent studies suggest that the chance for college admission may be lessened among high school seniors who are obese.

THE HEALTH RISKS

Almost every medical scientist in the country agrees that there are serious health hazards associated with obesity: increased risk of stroke, diabetes, high blood pressure; and diseases of the heart, blood vessels, liver, kidneys, and gallbladder. In addition, obesity can contribute to menstrual disorders, complications during pregnancy, and certain forms of arthritis. Too much weight overburdens the bones and joints, and can interfere with proper functioning of the lungs. There is also an increased risk of emphysema. Occasionally, the lack of proper air intake even threatens brain function. In short, all that extra fat stuffed in and around every organ and muscle places added stress on every part of the body. The well-known Framingham Study, a comprehensive investigation of cardiovascular diseases within a particular community, has pointed out the increased mortality rates for persons who are substantially above (or below) their Desirable Weight.

If you now happen to be only mildly overweight, none of these dangers apply to you. But we are compelled to remind you that a mere fifty excess calories per day over ten years' time will increase your weight by fifty pounds. As more weight is added, activity becomes more laborious and tends to decline; as the body becomes more sedentary, still more weight is added. Furthermore, after conducting extensive research on obesity, physicians at the Mayo Clinic report that repeated dieting is in itself a health hazard, and that repeated rapid changes in weight increase the risk of coronary heart disease.

68

The good news is that, with *permanent* weight loss, most of these hazards are reversible. (The major exception is emphysema. Once that disease has been contracted, it doesn't disappear, no matter what the size of your waistline.) Mortality rates for normal-weight men who were once obese are about the same as for those who were never obese. So if you have a weight problem, you owe it to yourself and your family to do something about it—right now.

OBESITY AND QUACKERY

At one time or another, most people try to "do something" about their weight. What many of them are doing is investing in useless diet books and other forms of nonsense.

Forever in search of an easy-off method, most overweight people will try almost anything that doesn't sound too much like a reducing diet. (As Ronald Deutsch notes in *The New Nuts Among the Berries,* "diet" is a four-letter word.) Countless authors have discovered just how well fad-diet books sell, and some of them have realized enormous profits. We discussed the actual dollar estimates for Dr. Robert Atkins' *Diet Revolution* in chapter 1. This book is typical of many. A number of women's magazines regularly feature new diets, sometimes monthly, and frequently help to promote diet books by offering their own condensed versions. Recently, a few men's business magazines have also taken up the craze.

In addition to diets, there are the health spas, or, to be less euphemistic, the "fat farms." Other approaches include reducing clinics, some legitimate, some not; and more kinds of exercise machines and garments than it seems conceivable the wildest of imaginations could dream up. And we can add to these the many, many pseudo-nutritionists who consult (for a fee!) and people like the late Adelle Davis, who once told a magazine interviewer, "Obese people are obese because they're getting so few nutrients to build energy to keep fat worked off."

What this all amounts to, of course, is Big Business. Whichever way the overweight person turns, someone is ready, waiting to pounce and exploit, to take advantage of the average American's lack of willpower, not to mention his gullibility. In *FDA Consumer* (March 1978), Nancy Glick reported that every year an estimated 70 million or more Americans spend upward of $10 billion on diet books, antiobesity prescriptions, over-the-counter appetite suppressants, reducing pills, diuretics, mechanical reducing devices, health spas, and special diets. And this number has no doubt increased appreciably since 1978.

By definition, a fad diet is one that differs substantially from a normal balanced diet. Fortunately, for that reason alone, few people find it feasible to follow such a regimen for any length of time. The more extreme a diet is, the greater is its threat to health. Those who have no medical problems other than obesity are not too likely to suffer any *permanent* effects from a few weeks of fad eating, but anything longer than that could spell big trouble. Borderline medical conditions might be precipitated, and existing conditions might be aggravated.

The object of any reducing diet is to take off excess weight and keep it off, not to torment your body to a point that jeopardizes health. Unfortunately, not enough people are able to distinguish between diets that can safely reduce poundage and those that merely reduce the size of their wallets. We'll take a look at a few of them to give you an idea of what to *avoid*.

Background Basics

First, however, we want to acquaint you briefly with a few simple nutritional facts. Read them carefully. They will help you to judge for yourself which kinds of diets are safe and may be effective, and which ones defy the laws of logic.

(1) A calorie is a measurement of energy. Physicists use this term to refer to a very small amount of energy. In nutrition, we talk about a different, larger calorie. Technically, the nutritionist's calorie is a kilocalorie; it's equal to one thousand of

the physicist's little calories. The nutritionist's calorie is sometimes called a large calorie, and it may be written with a capital C in technical nutrition books. In this book, when we use the term calorie, we're always referring to the large calorie used in nutrition.

(2) To maintain weight, calories in must equal calories out. That is, the number of calories expended in physical activity and normal body maintenance must be the same as the number of calories ingested in the form of food and beverages. If you eat and drink more than you burn up, you will gain weight; if you burn up more than you eat and drink, you will lose weight. When we say "drink," we mean calorie-containing beverages. Some of these drinks provide us with calories from sugar and alcohol, while others, especially milk, provide protein and several vitamins and minerals.

(3) A pound of body fat equals approximately 3,500 calories. Therefore, if you eat 500 calories per day below the number you expend in energy, you will lose one pound of fat by the end of a week (500 × 7). If, in addition, you burn up an additional 500 calories per day in the form of exercise, you will lose two pounds of fat after one week. (Diets claiming weight loss of two or three pounds or more a week should be viewed with suspicion for two reasons: First, food intake may be so limited as to jeopardize nutritional health if continued for any substantial length of time; second, a large proportion of any weight reduction in the first week or so would be due to water loss rather than body fat.)

(4) A gram of dietary fat contains 9 calories—more than twice as many as either proteins or carbohydrates, each of which contain 4 calories per gram. (Alcohol hovers near the middle at 7 calories per gram.) Vitamins, water, fiber, and minerals contain no calories.

(5) While it is obvious that fatty foods and alcoholic beverages should be cut back if you're trying to lose weight, no one should attempt to eliminate *all* fat from the diet, nor is it necessary to eliminate all alcoholic beverages. Some fat is essential

for good health. Fat performs many functions in the body (for instance, the transportation of fat-soluble vitamins like A and D). Further, it provides satiety value at mealtime; or, in other words, a reasonable amount of fat is what allows us to feel comfortably "full" after eating. The common observation that one is hungry again an hour after eating a Chinese dinner is explained by the low fat content of many Oriental dishes. If you're trying to eat less, you won't want too many meals that leave you feeling hungry again long before your next mealtime.

(6) Carbohydrates—sugars and starches—are often mistakenly accused of being the cause of overweight. Too many of them, like too many calories from any source, will put on pounds. But carbohydrates are vital to the diet. Deprivation causes headaches, weakness, lethargy, and dizziness, among other symptoms. The American Medical Association reports that fatigue is apparent after only two days on a very low carbohydrate diet. Additionally, an inadequate carbohydrate intake places an increased burden on the kidneys and favors an elevated blood-uric-acid level which can exacerbate gout. Low blood pressure (hypotension) frequently occurs in adults who eat carbohydrate-deficient diets and in unborn babies whose mothers are following this unwise dietary restriction. Beware of any diet advocating little or no sugar and starches. These are frequently the most popular, because reduced carbohydrate causes abnormally large water losses. And the scale then shows a concomitant weight loss, which most dieters mistakenly interpret as loss of body fat.

(7) Many fad diets appear to work for the first few days, because what the dieter is experiencing is primarily a loss of *water,* not fat, due to metabolic changes. But like a dried prune, when water levels are restored to normal, the body becomes plump and juicy again. Such diets also may work initially because most people who are fat *know* they eat too much. On a new diet they eat less, at least for a few days.

Diets Galore

The *Consumer Guide* book on dieting in 1980 (*Diets '80* by Theodore Berland, vol. 266, May 1980) rates over *eighty* different reducing diets. And that doesn't even include one we came across recently entitled *God's Answer to Fat* ("God wants to take away that fat appetite and give you a slender one.") The number alone should be sufficient proof that if any of them really worked, there wouldn't need to be so many.

DR. ATKINS' DIET REVOLUTION

Since we referred earlier to Dr. Robert Atkins, his first book seems a good place to begin.

Atkins is very fond of fat. In fact, he recommends that the simplest way to lose weight is to eat all you want of such dishes as eggs Benedict with hollandaise sauce, lobster Newburg, spareribs, roast pork—and lots of well-marbled steak. On the forbidden list are all carbohydrates, including, during the first phase of the diet, all fruits and vegetables (because they contain compounds known as complex carbohydrates).

High-fat diets have been around for over a century, so with even a modicum of honesty the regimen can hardly be dubbed "revolutionary." But Atkins has added his own twist. He professes to have discovered that when one consumes no carbohydrates, a "fat-mobilizing hormone" is secreted which converts the body from a carbohydrate-burning engine to a fat-burning engine. Just how the consumption of more fat stimulates the body to burn up its own stored fat is never made clear.

Atkins also promises that no one will feel hungry on such a diet, which is no doubt true. The calorie count is much too high. But the book is filled with misinformation and sheer nonsense, such as Atkins' contention that insulin is "the fattening hormone" and increases blood triglyceride (a type of fat) levels, and that sugar causes "basic metabolic disturbances" and B vitamin deficits.

Nationwide, *Dr. Atkins' Diet Revolution* has been criticized by legitimate nutritional scientists since its original publication in 1972. The American Medical Association's Council on Foods and Nutrition has expressed its "deep concern" and confirms that such a bizarre regimen is "without scientific merit." The chairman of the board of the New York County Medical Society said it was "unethical and self-aggrandizing." The list of similar statements is a long one. In 1973, the Senate Select Committee on Nutrition and Human Needs was prompted to conduct a hearing on Atkins' theories, with the outcome that the book's paperback publisher (Bantam) now includes a disclaimer in the front of the book. The committee and a host of medical authorities remain greatly disturbed by the hazards inherent in the Atkins diet: Fat and cholesterol levels are raised in the blood; heart disease may be aggravated by the metabolic disturbances; diarrhea is common on high-fat diets, with its accompanying loss of vitamins and minerals; and any or all of the dangers associated with low-carbohydrate diets, such as headaches, dizziness, and kidney problems, may occur. A pregnant woman following such a regimen is risking untold damage to her unborn baby.

The later book, *Dr. Atkins' Superenergy Diet,* merely expands his original statements to accommodate also those who are trying to maintain weight, put on weight, or cope with excess pounds during special circumstances like pregnancy; as well as anyone else who is looking for the "answer to fatigue and depression." Too few carbohydrates are *not* going to alleviate fatigue and depression—rather, they may aggravate both—and we have just observed that the diet can be disastrous during pregnancy. (In fact, no pregnant woman should follow *any* weight-reduction program. Pregnancy is a time for gaining some weight.) What it boils down to is anything *but* superenergy.

There is simply no way to consume all the high-calorie foods you wish, amounting to an average of perhaps 4,000–5,000 cal-

74

ories a day, and still lose weight. You may notice an initial weight loss, but this is chiefly water. The lack of carbohydrates makes the diet nutritionally inadequate, and it quickly becomes boring. The large amounts of fat are ultimately nauseating, so it might be possible to continue losing weight just from eating less, but this diet is a very wrong way to go about it. It is essentially a form of planned malnutrition.

Dr. Atkins' latest book is *Dr. Atkins' Nutritional Breakthrough: How to Treat Your Medical Condition Without Drugs.* The program incorporates the original diet and vitamin supplements for the treatment of insomnia, depression, alcoholism, headache, colds, cancer, arthritis, diabetes, atherosclerosis, hypertension, and more. For each particular ailment a vitamin and diet regimen is recommended. From this regimen Dr. Atkins predicts better health.

However, Dr. Atkins relies on highly questionable evidence to support his therapeutic claims. Sometimes the evidence is anecdotal, and sometimes it is simply incorrect.

Dr. Atkins claims that cholesterol is not a serious factor in the tendency toward heart disease. Further, he asserts that his high-fat diet actually reduces blood cholesterol levels. Another example: Atkins claims that his regimen will reduce the risk of diabetes by eliminating its frequent precursor, hypoglycemia. (To the contrary, there is much evidence suggesting that hypoglycemia is a rare disease, and that it is not associated with diabetes.) Atkins also attributes all depression and fatigue to hypoglycemia, even though their connection has not been well established. Perhaps Dr. Atkins' most revealing observation is that "laetrile is not controversial." He points to its therapeutic benefits. Unfortunately, he does not note the cyanide poisoning often associated with laetrile therapy. This omission is irresponsible.

Dr. Atkins' Nutrition Breakthrough is at best ineffective. At worst, it is dangerous because it advocates the disuse of potentially helpful drugs in the therapy of certain diseases. It also encourages the use of unproven agents as home remedies.

This kind of recommendation can lead to serious medical neglect.

Probably the best known of the late Dr. Irwin Stillman's books is *The Doctor's Quick Weight Loss Diet,* sometimes called the water diet, since it requires you to drink at least eight glasses of water per day (in addition to coffee, tea, and diet drinks in any amount desired).

Stillman's gimmick is protein. At some point in his career he came to believe that protein molecules are so large that extra energy is required to digest them. Thus, he has proposed that a low-fat, low-carbohydrate, high-protein diet will burn up an additional 275 calories per day; and that eating all you want of lean meat, poultry, fish, seafood, eggs, and low-fat cheeses will cause you to lose weight. No frying, and *no other foods* are allowed. All that water is necessary to rid the body of its partially burned fats, or ketones, to avoid bad breath and kidney irritation. Following Stillman's diet plan, a person would be permitted to consume as much cottage cheese and sour cream as desired, but not even one saltine cracker is allowed (i.e., you're permitted to eat five cups of cottage cheese for lunch which contain about 1,000 calories, but you cannot eat one cup of cottage cheese and two saltines which contain less than 250 calories).

Stillman's diets, like those of Atkins, violate one of the basic laws of thermodynamics, namely that energy doesn't just disappear. You need to be suspicious of any diet that allows "all you can eat" of any food that contains more than a few calories per serving. Also, the Stillman diet allows so few kinds of foods that it is impossible to get adequate amounts of all of the different nutrients required for good health. The main virtue of this regimen is that it is too monotonous for most people to stick with for very long. Yet in the ten years following the book's initial publication in 1967, it sold over five million copies—and it is still available in many bookstores.

THE SCARSDALE DIET

Another rehash of the high-protein, low-carbohydrate, low-fat diets is found in *The Complete Scarsdale Medical Diet Plus Dr. Tarnower's Lifetime Keep-Slim Program,* by the late Dr. Herman Tarnower and Samm Sinclair Baker (who also collaborated on Dr. Stillman's diet books). That's a rather long-winded title for so little useful information.

The "Medical" Diet promises to rid you of at least ten to fourteen pounds (perhaps as much as twenty) in two weeks. At the end of the two weeks comes a switch to the Keep-Slim Program for two more weeks. If there are still pounds to be shed, it's back for two more weeks on the Medical Diet. And so forth. The menu selections are explicit; practically no substitutions are allowed; there are no calories to count; and portion sizes are not indicated for meats, vegetables, or most fruits—only the admonition "not to overload the stomach." Now, that would be a reasonable suggestion, except that an inability to gauge stomach overload undoubtedly contributed to the overweight condition in the first place.

Consumer Guide magazine's evaluation: "Great Dr. Stillman's ghost." There is no more magic in the protein of the Scarsdale Diet than there is in the Stillman Diets. Tarnower has told us that his own is not a fad diet, a statement we find incomprehensible in view of its extreme rigidity and the fact that it is designed for only two weeks at a time.

LIQUID PROTEIN

The goal of any diet is learning to live *with* food, not without it. A weight-loss regimen that consists solely of a few daily doses of "liquid protein" accomplishes nothing toward the achievement of permanent weight control. What it does is to create a host of medical problems. (Note: Don't confuse liquid protein with liquid-formula diets, such as Metrecal. The latter are boring, and they teach the dieter nothing about good eating patterns, but

77

they are usually not medically dangerous. In some individuals, however, diarrhea and/or constipation may occur).

Consumer Guide reports that since the mid-seventies, as many as sixty deaths have been attributed to liquid-protein dieting. There is no way even to tabulate the disastrous—and sometimes irreversible—effects on the hearts, kidneys, and livers of countless other dieters. Many have contracted gallstones, kidney stones, gout, or ulcerative colitis, as well as developing numerous side effects like hair loss, muscle weakness, nausea, headaches, dizziness, bad breath, skin dryness, serious potassium imbalance, decreased sex drive, difficulty in keeping warm, menstrual irregularities, constipation, and nervous disorders. The extensive metabolic changes resulting from the "liquid-protein" diet also affect medication required for such chronic diseases as diabetes and high blood pressure.

The most highly publicized of the liquid-protein diets is *The Last Chance Diet,* summarized in a 1976 book of that name by osteopath Dr. Robert Linn. Linn's idea is that this "protein-sparing fast" offers all the advantages of total fasting (i.e., quick weight loss), while at the same time preventing the body from raiding its stores of protein from muscles and vital organs. In his book, Linn tells us that liquid protein provides a "safe, nutritional regimen." It is neither.

Linn's protein was originally called Prolinn, but, to avoid legal entanglements, he was forced to publish the formula, with the result that a number of other manufacturers began marketing basically identical products under different brand names. None of them, without the addition of other food elements, provides adequate nutrition. The form of protein used in these formulas is hydrolyzed collagen, which lacks several of the essential amino acids. The recommended dose of liquid protein is equal to 60 grams of protein, or about 240 calories per day. Yet while the dieter's starved body struggles to digest that protein, it still must raid its own body protein, because the missing essential amino acids in this liquid-protein product prevent it from being used to preserve body protein tissue.

78

The collagen in Prolinn is derived from beef hides, sow underbelly, and animal hooves and horns, which are cooked in a broth with enzymes and tenderizers to break down the tissue. (The effect is a form of "predigestion.") The resulting gooey syrup is then spiked strongly with artificial fruit flavoring. Not only does the brew *sound* unappetizing, it has a history of being concocted under somewhat less than sanitary conditions. More than once in 1977, health authorities on both local and national levels found it necessary to confiscate contaminated supplies.

The Food and Drug Administration issued a new ruling, effective in August 1980, that all protein supplements (liquid or powder) used in reducing diets must carry the following label:

Warning—Very low-calorie protein diets (below 800 Calories per day) may cause serious illness or death. Do not use for weight reduction without medical supervision. Use with particular care if you are taking medication. Not for use by infants, children, or pregnant or nursing women.

According to the *Federal Register* (April 4, 1980), the FDA found that protein-diet-related deaths apparently had little direct connection with the quality of the protein, but that the symptomatic patterns were "highly suggestive of death by starvation." Consequently, the FDA warns against *any* very low-calorie diet—that is, any diet below 800 calories per day.

But bookstores continue to sell *The Last Chance Diet*. Drugstores continue to sell liquid and powdered protein (good money-makers, since vitamin/mineral supplements can usually be peddled at the same time). And Dr. Linn continues to operate his string of diet clinics (which *U.S. News and World Report* stated in late 1977 were extracting sixty dollars per patient for each required weekly visit). Since Linn also warns that the diet requires medical supervision, his clinics thrive. But the real concern here is for the rest of the liquid-protein dieters who will continue to ignore Linn's admonishment, as well as the label warnings, and thus remain unaware of adverse changes that may be occurring within themselves.

Linn's promise of a twenty-to-twenty-five-pound weight loss during the first month is tempting. But starvation is a hazardous and thus foolish form of self-punishment.

Another very low-calorie formula diet is the Cambridge Diet. It was developed in Cambridge, England, by a team of British researchers. One great advantage it has over The Last Chance Diet is that it has good nutritional quality protein, namely milk and soya protein, and is fortified with several vitamins and minerals, including potassium and magnesium. It is available in powdered form and easily mixed with hot or cold water. It is also available in a variety of soups and puddings. The initial recommended daily dosage provides only 330 calories, 33 grams of protein, 3 grams of fat, the remainder being carbohydrate.

The Cambridge Diet has been well tested in a variety of hospital and research studies, but in our opinion it is a dangerous diet to follow for any length of time unless one is either in a hospital or under careful and frequent medical supervision.

Here are some of the comments of the American Dietetic Association on the Cambridge Diet Plan. "It should be a real money-maker. And it promises to give dietitians another problem to wrestle with. The dieting begins with the Cambridge Formula powder—the 'Ultimate Diet, a complete and delicious food that actually melts off fat virtually as rapidly as complete fasting.'

". . . If you have only a few pounds to lose, it is suggested that you stay on the formula for at least a week and go immediately to the Add-A-Meal Interval, and then progress onto your Lifetime Nutrition Program. If you have a large number of pounds to lose, you stay on the Cambridge Diet four weeks and then switch immediately to the Add-A-Meal Interval for seven to ten days. If you have achieved your desired body weight by then, you can go on to the Lifetime Nutrition Program. . . .

"You then continue back and forth, four weeks Cambridge Diet and seven to ten days Add-A-Meal Interval, until you achieve your weight-loss goals. The brochure describing the diet promises that the Cambridge Add-A-Meal Interval and the Cambridge Lifetime Nutrition Program from the Cambridge Kitchen will help keep you slim and trim forever. Cambridge has developed 400-, 200-, 100-, and 50-calorie 'Cambridge Crown' recipes that not only are delicious but also provide the proper balance of carbohydrate to protein, to fat, so that you can continue to enjoy balanced nutrition. And so on—with Cambridge Mini-Exercise Program."

The Cambridge Diet, like all liquid diets, does nothing to train the dieter in new eating habits, and thus, after a period of time, one will usually rapidly regain any weight lost on such a low-calorie diet.

A very undesirable and dangerous feature of the Cambridge Diet is that it is largely distributed by door-to-door sales personnel referred to as Cambridge Counselors. We would have to question whether many of these "counselors" are qualified to give medical advice, supervision, or to assist and follow through to see that the individual does receive proper medical supervision. After all, most qualified health professionals would recognize the dangers of this diet and, therefore, not be so anxious to advocate its use.

THE SIMEONS HCG DIET

HCG is Human Chorionic Gonadotropin, a growth hormone secreted by the placenta which can be extracted from the urine of pregnant women. Dr. Albert T. Simeons first used HCG in the treatment of young boys suffering from a condition known as Froehlich's Syndrome. Injections of the hormone helped reduce the accumulation of feminizing fat on the hips, buttocks, and thighs, which had made such boys look somewhat feminine.

Simeons and his followers then reasoned that with the liberated fat as a major source of nourishment, dieters could also benefit from the drug.

Thus began the chain of Simeons Weight Reduction Institutes which quickly spread across the country. (Simeons has also written a book, called *Pounds and Inches—A New Approach to Obesity*.) By 1974 lawsuits were not uncommon, as the realization grew that many of the so-called clinics were being operated by lay businessmen who paid certain doctors large sums to refer patients to the HCG program. Studies by the Food and Drug Administration concluded that "there are no scientifically adequate, well-controlled clinical studies appearing in medical literature which establish the safety and efficacy of HCG in the treatment of obesity."

The HCG treatment is accompanied by a diet of only 500 calories a day, so inevitably the dieter will lose weight. No fat is allowed, and the only cosmetics permitted are rouge, lipstick, and eyebrow pencil, in keeping with Simeons' peculiar theory that any oils applied to the skin will be absorbed into the body to add to fat stores. A diet that is very low in calories carries hazards of its own, but the additional deliberate exposure to the unknown, possibly long-term effects of such a potent hormone as HCG is just not advisable.

DR. FRANK'S NO-AGING DIET

Since its publication in 1976, Dr. Benjamin S. Frank's book has become a favorite with all those in search of the Fountain of Youth. "Eat and grow younger," Frank urges us, by eating foods that are rich in the nucleic acids RNA and DNA. What that seems to translate into is lots of sardines. Three days a week he allows seafood other than sardines, and once a week a special treat of calves' liver. Lots of beets (or borscht), soybeans, and lentils are good; and he recommends such other universal favorites as chicken hearts, oysters, squid, asparagus, and radishes. Frank insists there are no firm "don'ts" but then goes on to comment on the shortcomings of almost everything most of us are used to eating.

Frank's great "scientific breakthrough of our age" is supposed to make every cell in our bodies young again. His theory is that since RNA and DNA (nucleic acids containing the components essential for several enzyme reactions necessary for replacing

82

worn-out cells with new ones) are scientifically accepted as the fundamental genetic material that determines the essential makeup of each living creature, increased consumption of these vital compounds will inhibit the degenerative changes of the aging process. Not only will sardine eaters *look* younger, but, claims Frank, chronic diseases of the elderly can be avoided or alleviated.

All of that is couched in a great deal of scientific-sounding jargon and gobbledygook. The problem is that it only *sounds* scientific. Nothing in any field of science even suggests that our bodies benefit from consumption of extra nucleic acids. They are broken down in digestion, like all other substances, and then remade into needed compounds.

The particularly ludicrous part of Frank's theory totally ignored in his book is the fact that genetic material is extremely specific. If the nucleic acids of a sardine were to have any direct effect on our bodies, about the most we could expect would be to grow fins and improve our swimming!

This extreme diet would particularly endanger the health of anyone with hypertension, because of the high salt content of the sardines; and of those with gout, because foods rich in RNA and DNA have a high purine content—a specific compound involved in gout.

When *Family Circle* ran its adaptation of *Dr. Frank's No-Aging Diet,* considerable attention was devoted to Dr. Sheldon Hendler's introduction to the book. The magazine identified him as a University of California professor. Yet when William K. Stuckey was researching his *New York* magazine article about the book, he attempted to locate Hendler, only to discover that he had never been a professor at any University of California campus, although he had once been employed there as a part-time tutor. Contrary to all the wonderful things Hendler originally said about the book, what he eventually told Stuckey is highly enlightening: "Who the hell knows whether Frank's diet is a no-aging diet? I just wanted to help the old guy out. . . . He's in great health but a little on the crazy side, and what the hell, he may be right about nucleic acids. . . . Sardines? I haven't the slightest idea why he stresses them so. Maybe he just likes sardines."*

What Stuckey and others have found utterly appalling is the editors' own admission that no attempt was made by either Dial Press (the book's publisher) or *Family Circle* to contact established scientific authorities in order to verify the logic of Frank's theory or to determine the diet's safety.†

As appealing as the no-aging theory may sound to many, the verdict is neatly summarized by noted nutritionist Dr. Harold A. Harper, dean of graduate studies at the University of California (San Francisco): "This diet is absolute, sheer quackery. I repeat that statement. It is totally unscientific from A to Z. To anyone who knows the remotest thing about chemistry, [Frank's] theory reads like a comic book."

THE EASY NO-FLAB DIET

Dr. Richard Passwater, who in the past has showered the public with misinformation in the form of such publications as *Supernutrition: Megavitamin Revolution* and *Supernutrition for Healthy Hearts,* has augmented this nonsense with his 1979 book, *The Easy No-Flab* (or FLAB) *Diet.* Passwater claims that dieters can lose weight only by counting FLAB units, an acronym for Fat Liquidating Ability Barometer, and has drawn up an elaborate FLAB index of common foods. "The body doesn't handle food in terms of calories," he tells us. "It handles food in terms of protein quality, carbohydrate quality, and fat quality." Thus, according to Passwater, although a four-ounce hamburger and a serving of two doughnuts each have

---

* It is worth noting that Frank's diet presented an obviously ideal opportunity for the sardine industry to realize a sharp increase in sales. However, the public-relations representative of the Norwegian sardine industry, Botsford Ketchum, and Vice-President Bee Marks stated that their client realized that endorsing a nutritionally unsound program would be an irresponsible, although profitable, disservice to the consumer. We applaud their excellent judgment.

† William K. Stuckey, "The 'No-Aging' Diet: Something Fishy Here," *New York,* October 11, 1976.

about the same number of calories (250), the doughnuts have 382 FLAB units, while the hamburger has only 177 and so is less fattening.

The manner by which FLAB units are calculated isn't terribly clear, rendering the diet impossible to follow without purchasing Passwater's $9.95 book. His idea has something to do with each food's alleged fat-storing or fat-burning properties, and the amount of insulin each causes to be released into the blood-stream.

Any diet that ignores the basic and universal nutritional principle of "calories in vs. calories out" is absurd. Perhaps as a consolation prize, Passwater offers a method for appetite control that involves applying finger pressure to one of two spots near the ears—a sort of "acupuncture-without-needles" technique, he tells us. That sounds suspiciously as though it might be more effective among cultures of alien beings who eat with their ears.

THE GRAPEFRUIT DIETS

The original "Grapefruit Diet" was another name for the so-called "Mayo Diet," which has never been in any way connected with the Mayo Clinic in Rochester, Minnesota. (The clinic does have a weight-reducing diet, but it is a sensible, nutritionally balanced one.)

The first Grapefruit Diet included only grapefruit and black coffee. Then came grapefruit, eggs, and bacon—naturally, all you could eat. Gradually, the various versions grew less restrictive as myths spread about the magical properties of grapefruit itself, until eventually the only requirement was that each meal begin with half a grapefruit. Apparently, dieters had deluded themselves into believing the fruit was a big yellow spark plug that would ignite their excess fat and cause it mysteriously to vanish.

Grapefruit is a fine food to include in a weight-reduction effort. It is relatively low in calories and contributes a substantial amount of vitamin C, as well as smaller amounts of other nutrients. That's all it is. It possesses no special powers that will wondrously burn away fat. But hoaxes die hard. The last few years have seen the development of various "grapefruit" pills, which are alleged to perform all the sorcery of real grapefruit without the necessity of even having to eat it.

THE HIGH FIBER / BRAN DIETS

Fiber is that part of foods that cannot be digested or absorbed by our bodies. It used to be referred to as "roughage." Many vegetables and the skins of fruits such as plums, grapes, and apples are high in fiber. There are several different kinds of fiber. Bran is the fiber in whole wheat products. Bran-containing foods may be helpful to those suffering from constipation, but, like grapefruit, bran possesses no special properties to aid in weight loss—nor is it a cure-all means of disease control. As we saw in chapter 1, however, advocacy of the marvels of bran can be traced at least as far back as Sylvester Graham and his whole grain flour. No matter that scientists later disproved the notion that daily (or multidaily) bowel movements are necessary to keep the human body free of "poisons." As night follows day, modern crusaders eventually revived bran as the newest "wonder food."

Not too many years ago a group of British researchers, headed by Dr. Denis Burkitt and Dr. Hugh Trowel, attempted to discover why certain groups of African natives suffered so little diverticulitis, appendicitis, constipation, hemorrhoids, and colon cancer, compared to Europeans and North Americans. Their observations led to the hypothesis that the African high-fiber diet may be instrumental in keeping those populations lean and virtually free of many of the diseases of the intestine that are so common among us.

Although this has not been unequivocably proven, the theory was capitalized on by Dr. David Reuben in his 1975 book, *The Save-Your-Life Diet*. (In an earlier book, Reuben had already told the general populace everything they always wanted to know about sex but were afraid to ask, and more recently he is trying to tell them everything they "always wanted to know about nutrition"—but never will, if they depend on his book.) Reuben presents as proven fact the Burkitt and Trowel theory that bran

86

and other high-fiber foods offer protection from colon cancer, diverticulitis, and even heart disease. He prescribes a weight-reducing diet but does not specify any amounts of food except bran. And the amount of bran that Dr. Reuben recommends is not based on substantial scientific evidence. Nowhere in his book does he mention the fact that one of the primary reasons few Africans in the study groups suffer from some of the diseases he discusses is that they simply don't live long enough to develop them.

Notwithstanding, Dr. Sanford Siegal (an osteopath) climbed on the bran wagon and wrote his *Natural Fiber Permanent Weight Loss Diet.* Says Siegal, "Fiber will decrease the transit time of food through the intestinal tract, thus lowering the number of calories your body receives from the food you eat." He further claims that eating "fiber-free processed foods ... is the main cause of obesity in our society," and that by eating bran at every meal and eliminating refined carbohydrates we can remain slim forever. He, like Reuben, insists that bran and other fiber-containing foods help prevent diseases of the heart and colon.

In February 1980, the Sunday newspaper supplement, *Family Weekly,* which is part of hundreds of Sunday newspapers around the country, carried a full-page mail-order ad for something called *The Bran Diet,* published by U.S. Book Publishing Company but apparently authorless. The claims were even more extravagant than either Reuben's or Siegal's, asserting that cholesterol levels "which go with heart, lung, kidney, and artery disease are lowered astonishingly by dietary bran." It further promised to alleviate phlebitis and hemorrhoids, and to "mobilize the fat" from your body because "your body absorbs fewer calories than the same amount of regular food."*

No studies of either animals or Americans on high-fiber diets have yet shown that they develop any chronic diseases with less frequency than do those following medium-fiber diets. Nor are

---

* It is worth noting that during the same month the same supplement carried a similar ad for *The Rice Diet,* by the same publisher at the same price. The ad included many of the same claims and a major portion of *identically worded copy.*

there any indications that the increased speed of food passing through the digestive tract has anything to do with losing weight. What may be of greater concern is that some fiber is found in association with a substance known as phytic acid, which binds with iron, calcium, zinc, and perhaps other minerals, decreasing their absorption from the intestine and possibly leading to deficiencies. For that reason alone, unusually high-fiber diets over time could be undesirable.

A shift toward more high-fiber foods like vegetables and fruits may be beneficial to anyone who is trying to lose weight or who is constipated, in part because of the fiber, but also because vegetables and fruits are largely water and hence low in calories. But while bran-food products in small amounts are wholesome and delicious, don't overdo! (And don't expect miracles.) Warns Dr. Peter G. Lindner, a respected physician, "Fiber is just one part of a properly balanced diet. Undue emphasis on fiber, and especially adding it as a *food supplement* (e.g., bran) to an otherwise poor diet, will probably cause more problems than it solves." (Italics his.)

THE NEW CARBOHYDRATE AND GRAM COUNTER

This book by Margaret Sullivan currently graces the shelves of almost every store that sells books, however small the selection. Sullivan claims we can eat all the protein and fat we want and still lose weight, if we don't consume more than 60 grams of carbohydrate. That translates to 240 calories of carbohydrate and—presumably—anywhere up to 50,000 calories of everything else, if we so desire.

We won't insult our readers' intelligence by expounding on the obvious fallacies presented in that one.

THE ZEN MACROBIOTIC DIET

For some inane reason this regimen continues to be a favorite among certain members of the younger generation. "Macrobiotic" translates to a "long life," but strict adherence to the Zen

Macrobiotic Diet can mean precisely the opposite. A number of tragic deaths by starvation on this diet have been reported, and the cases of resulting malnutrition are legion.

The diet's popularity is evidently due in part to the mistaken idea that it is an outgrowth of Zen Buddhism. In fact, there is no connection; true Buddhists find food faddism abhorrent. Nevertheless, the diet employs a mixture of occultism, mysticism, and dietary extremism in its promise to cure all illness, past and present (including such conditions as epilepsy), while at the same time offering to improve memory and judgment and "expand freedom and thinking." Its followers believe that everything in the world is part of "yin" and "yang," and that healthy eating should offer a ratio of five yin to one yang. Sugar and most fruits are too yin and must be limited; meats and eggs are too yang; and the only perfect food is brown rice. (Believe it or not, this is not an exaggeration of the diet's claims. People follow this diet religiously.)

The Zen Macrobiotic Diet is actually a series of diets. The lowest level still retains some semblance of balance, even though it prohibits many common foods such as citrus fruits, potatoes, and milk products. The seventh (in some versions, the tenth) and highest level, however, is retricted to brown rice and limited amounts of fluid, usually tea. Such a diet is deficient in most nutrients, including calories and water.

Next to prolonged total fasting, this diet is probably the most dangerous fad diet in existence.

THE CRENSHAW SUPER BEAUTY DIET

This diet is notable only in that so many other fad diets have been patterned after one or more of its "miracle" ingredients: kelp, lecithin, cider vinegar, and vitamin B_6. Mary Ann Crenshaw calls these her "Four Friends" and first introduced them to the public in 1974, via *Family Circle* magazine and her book, *The Natural Way to Super Beauty*. Crenshaw's prescription will help you lose weight *only* if you also follow a low-calorie diet as she recommends. The rest of it is nonsense. To wit:

Kelp (a kind of seaweed) is beneficial, according to Crenshaw, because its iodide content stimulates the thyroid and leads to stepped-up metabolism and subsequent weight loss. Fact: The human body gets more than sufficient iodide through the consumption of seafood and/or iodized salt. Furthermore, excessive amounts of this mineral can have the opposite effect, depressing the thyroid and thus slowing metabolism.

About lecithin: Crenshaw says to "pronounce it 'less-i-thin' and call it a miracle." In fact, this substance actually *aids* absorption of dietary fat in the intestine. Thus, it tends to increase the fat calories available to the body. This contradicts any claims made for its promotion of weight loss. In any case, the human body produces its own lecithin and does not require supplements.

A teaspoon of cider vinegar in a glass of water is advised after every meal (à la Dr. D. C. Jarvis of folk-medicine fame). Crenshaw's theory is that since oil and vinegar don't mix, fat and vinegar won't mix either, and "vinegar just might win out."

Vitamin B_6, also known as pyridoxine, is included in the diet in order to help burn away the fat—a strange conclusion, indeed, in view of the fact that the major functions of B_6 involve the breakdown and utilization of proteins. Scientists are unsure whether this vitamin has *any* function in relation to fat.

You can safely skip taking supplements of all four of Crenshaw's "friends." None will have the least effect on your size, shape, or state of health (with the possible exception of iodide overdose), and you will get plenty of their nutrients in any diet selected from the Basic Four Food Groups.

A FEW OF THE EVEN MORE SILLY DIETS

There are so many of these it has been difficult to decide which to include in a small amount of space. For starters, there's the Lollipop Diet, which recommends lollipops in place of higher-calorie snack foods. Then there's the Holy Cow Diet, which allows no beef. *The Hollywood Emergency Diet,* by actor Frank Downing, makes much of the use of fructose (also known as fruit sugar) instead of other forms of sugar. Additional weight-loss weapons, he tells us, are brewer's yeast and those "old friends," lecithin and kelp.

Then along came the Diet of the Desperate Housewife. (Not only does its title sound like a mystery, why it would work is even more so.) This one was presented by Nancy Pryor, author-publisher of *The Amazing Diet Secret of a Desperate Housewife.* Amazing, indeed! Pryor, like Downing, is evidently completely lacking in any knowledge of basic biochemistry. Her first group of "secrets" involves the use of fructose, which, she instructs us, is to be eaten before each meal, because "it can be assimilated directly into your muscle cells" and it "raises your blood sugar level without inducing an insulin reponse." In actual fact, fructose—like every other carbohydrate—is converted by the body into glucose or blood sugar (the energy source for the entire body, including the brain). Pryor also recommends dieting every other day and taking regular supplements of—are you ready?—lecithin, kelp, brewer's yeast, dolomite, yogurt, and wheat germ.

The diet parade continues with those that advise us to "count bites, not calories"; "give your appetite to Jesus"; "think yourself a perfect figure"; and "nibble the fat away." Back in the 1930s, there was even a "gargle your fat away" diet. That one employed the use of Helen's Liquid Reducer Compound, which chemical analysis eventually revealed to be merely peppermint-flavored hydrogen peroxide. About that same time, however, thyroid shots also became popular, under the theory that the resulting stepped-up metabolism would burn away fat more readily. But beware! A few unscrupulous doctors still use this method of treating obese patients, even though they must know that administration of thyroid hormone can be extremely dangerous to the heart and other organs by causing the entire body to work overtime.

THE "BEVERLY HILLS" DIET

Of the seven diet books that were on the 1981 *New York Times* best-seller list, *The Beverly Hills Diet* was number one. Since then, its monetary success has been rivaled only by author Judy Mazel's ignorance of nutrition. She is an ex-showbiz diet experimenter who contrived the diet (by trial and error) for her own 170-pound body. Finding it personally effective, she decided to write a book to "make the world slim" and "put a smile on people's faces." Instead of smiles, however, Mazel has created a dangerous nutritional regimen.

The diet is based on the fictional nutritional principle that certain foods in combination can clog your stomach's enzyme system and keep food from being properly digested. As a result, it turns into fat. She notes that "fruits should be eaten alone or else they get trapped by other foods in your stomach." Along the same lines, proteins should be eaten only with other proteins, and carbohydrates with other carbohydrates, or possibly fats.

Mazel's enzyme system consists of ptyalin, hydrochloric acid (which is not an enzyme), and pepsin. She attributes the digestion of carbohydrate to ptyalin, the digestion of protein to pepsin, and the digestion of fat to HCL. (Never mind the well-established fact that bile helps to digest fat, and that digestion occurs mostly in the small intestine through the actions of hundreds of enzymes.) She claims that the few enzymes she mentions work against each other and result in inefficient digestion. Here is Judy Mazel's description of carbohydrate and protein eaten in "mis" combination: "The stomach gets frustrated and says, 'What am I going to do with you?' And here the carb stays festering, fermenting ... ultimately turning to fat." The notion that undigested food transforms into fat is without any scientific basis. Undigested food is eliminated from the body.

Mazel's great elixir is fruit. She believes that pineapples, strawberries, papayas, mangoes, kiwis, and persimmons contain the enzymes used in the stomach's digestive process. Consequently, they are absorbed into the system and "burn up fat." This is voodoo unknown to physiology. Our body enzymes are made internally, mostly by the pancreas and small intestine. All enzymes are proteins and all proteins ingested, including "fatburning" enzymes, are broken down by most cooking procedures or by the hydrochloric acid in the stomach, and rendered completely inactive. The enzymes in the food we eat do not in any way increase those available for digestive purposes.

The Beverly Hills explanation of diet and nutrition would be amusing were it not for the fact that Mazel applies it to a diet she calls "healthy." For the first week or ten days of the Beverly Hills Diet, the dieter eats only fruit. (Actually, with the exception of three and a half bagels, corn on the cob, and two potatoes.)

There are no representatives from the milk group, because Mazel says milk is good for growth and adults don't need it. In reality, milk is the main source of body calcium and phosphorus, needed for bone maintenance and repair. It is also an excellent source of protein. There are no representatives from the meat group, which also supplies nutritionally complete protein, the element most severely missing from the Beverly Hills Diet. According to the regimen, there is very little protein until the end of the third week. Such protein deprivation can result in a myriad of bodily malfunctions, particularly diarrhea, which is admittedly a good (albeit unhealthful and unpleasant) way to lose weight. Lack of dietary protein can also cause the breakdown of lean body mass (another term for body protein), resulting in a concomitant loss of potassium. Low potassium leads to muscular weakness, respiratory problems, renal disorders, and potential cardiac irregularity. There are no representatives from the cereal group in the Mazel diet either, and although carbohydrates are supplied by the fruit, these fruits are not good sources of niacin, iron, thiamine, riboflavin, and dozens of other necessary nutrients. (But Judy Mazel says, "So if one day out of their lives they might be a little short of niacin—so what?") There is, however, an overwhelming supply of fiber and vitamin C.

The first and second weeks, in conclusion, are a nutritional disaster. Weeks three through six add more foods, but the diet is still low in protein, calcium, thiamine, riboflavin, and niacin.

It is not a surprise that this diet causes weight loss. The average daily caloric intake is about 500 calories. Also, on this regimen true weight loss will be accompanied by a substantial water weight loss. The overall result will be fewer pounds, but poorer health.

Judy Mazel did not stop with a weight-loss book but continues spreading her hogwash in a new book describing how to maintain slimness throughout your lifetime. She calls her book, *The Beverly Hills Diet Lifetime Plan,* and claims that it will lead you into the "land of eternal slimhood." The book promulgates the same type of nonsense as the weight-loss book. Mazel still advocates eating only certain foods together and includes a number of recipes to help work this out. As with the first, this maintenance diet is *not* balanced and cannot be considered safe.

Mazel begins her book by trying to defend herself against criticism of the first diet, but such protestations do not make her diet any the less dangerous, nor do they provide any rationale for the maintenance program.

THE I LOVE NEW YORK DIET

New York is the center of the advertising business, so perhaps it should come as no surprise to find a lot of ad-style hype in the *I Love New York Diet* book. Readers are told that the diet "means a sexier you," and that "you'll find it a pleasure" to be on the diet, which "gives you a sense of well-being, vigor, and a peace of mind that you never experienced before." This is about as believable as a TV commercial.

Unfortunately, the book's claim that you'll "lose ten pounds in seven days" is also hype. Unless you're the size of King Kong and in training for the Olympics, no diet can accomplish that—at least not without a dangerously extreme reduction in calories. The I Love New York Diet is not that extreme (or dangerous).

The I Love New York Diet bears an uncanny resemblance to its suburban neighbor from Scarsdale. It includes a rigid crash diet and more moderate maintenance programs. The crash diet is very explicit, although (as with the Scarsdale Diet) no portion sizes are specified. Also, the diet tries to be low-fat and low-carbohydrate at the same time. This means that it is high in protein, but there is no more magic to protein in the big city than there was in Scarsdale.

The "crash program" of the I Love New York Diet is very heavy on vegetables and meat/poultry/fish. To lose weight effectively, the New York dieter should be careful about the portion sizes of the main dishes, since these animal foods pack a substantial calorie wallop. Some milk, breads, and cereals are included, so the diet isn't a nutritional disaster, but it's not magic, either. You could lose weight just as effectively on a less rigid diet that provided the same number of calories from a wider variety of foods.

As much as we love New York, we really can't recommend this diet. It promises too much more than it can deliver. If, however, you're trying to keep your weight down, rather than take some off, you might want to take a look at this book. There is a lot of good sense in the sections on weight maintenance and some mouth-watering low-calorie ethnic recipes. Unfortunately, though, the recipes are presented without calorie counts!

NEVER-SAY-DIET BOOK

Hurrah for a diet program that concentrates on changing eating habits, promoting exercise, and fostering the nutritional benefits of a diet based on the Basic Four Food Groups. Richard Simmons' *Never-Say-Diet Book* is a responsible guide to weight reduction.

A very small portion of the book is actually devoted to the diet. The regimen is listed in a few pages. The dieter is given a choice from columns A, B, and C for the day's menus. Consequently, variations are numerous. No single food group is emphasized over any other, and the meals are well balanced.

The diet has been dubbed a "volume" food plan, which simply means that Simmons encourages people to eat less of a variety of foods. As he says, "To have a healthy body—and a thin one— you need to eat a proper balance of foods that will keep you in perfect harmony."

95

Simmons calls his *Never-Say-Diet Book* a live-it book, because
a crucial part of the program is a reevaluation of mental attitudes
toward eating. Simmons uses quizzes and games to make the
dieter aware of poor food habits. He also provides encouragement and amusement with stories of his own dieting experience.
Simmons stresses the very sensible point that if you cannot control your appetite, no diet can do it for you; and that a permanent
weight loss can result only from a permanent change in the
amount and types of food eaten.

The live-it program also includes a schedule of simple exercises. No health clubs or equipment are required.

Finally, Simmons stresses communication with a physician
and a regular referral to his medical checklist.

OTHER GIMMICKS

The overweight person who is not yet convinced that eating
smaller quantities while maintaining a balanced diet is the only
safe and effective way to lose weight still has a choice of other
gimmicks. To judge from the abundance of advertisements in
magazines, tabloid newspapers, and Sunday supplements, a current favorite must be the various types of exercise suits and reducing-pajamas that are meant to sleep your fat away. Advertisements for one of these, marketed under the name Slim Sleepers,
insist that you will "wake up thinner than you were the night
before"; and the customer is invited to wear them for jogging,
cleaning house, and working in the yard. (The ads do not mention whether the garment is also suitable for the grocery store or
office, but it is reinforced with double seams.) In fact, all these
garments do is make you sweat more (which should give you an
idea of the discomfort involved), causing a temporary loss of
water weight.

Exercise machines are also widely advertised, but, having been
around for a while, their appeal is probably somewhat less novel.
The type that does all the work for you (vibrating belts, etc.) is
worthless. If it's *you* who does the exercising, with a device such

as a stationary bicycle (not operated by electricity), then you can actually burn up some calories. But most people have access to cheaper and more effective means of exercise. A daily brisk walk, for instance, is an excellent (and free) form of exercise. If you feel you *must* invest in a gadget, consider the virtues of a good jump rope. It costs only a few dollars and is an excellent way to firm up muscles.

Diet pills in enormous variety are promoted and marketed almost everywhere. Many of the over-the-counter variety are virtually useless. However, the FDA recently declared two ingredients in nonprescription diet pills, phenylpropanolamine (PPA) and benzocaine, to be "safe and effective." Going back to the laws of conservation of energy for a minute, you should realize that diet pills, even if the government swears by them, do not take off weight by themselves. All they can do is possibly reduce your appetite and thus help you stay on a low-calorie reducing diet. These pills, at best, are only a temporary crutch. They do not help in adjusting eating habits for maintaining a reduced weight. They are relatively safe, if used properly, and dangerous when taken improperly.

Benzocaine is a local anaesthetic that dulls the taste buds and presumably discourages eating. PPA, according to its manufacturers, is helpful in diet pills because it depresses the brain's "appetite center." However, it is unsafe for anyone who has heart disease, hypertension, diabetes, or thyroid disease. Since these conditions are common in overweight people, you should check with your doctor before trying PPA pills. If your doctor gives you an OK and you want to try them, you should take the following precautions: 1) Use the pills in combination with a sensible weight-loss diet; and 2) make sure you aren't taking any other nonprescription remedies containing the same ingredients. This is particularly important for PPA, which is also used as a nasal decongestant and is found in many brands of over-the-counter cold remedies. It is possible to get sick from excessive doses of

PPA, so you shouldn't be using two products that contain this ingredient at the same time. And certainly don't take PPA or any other alleged reducing pill if you are pregnant or trying to become pregnant.

As this book was being completed a new diet pill appeared, accompanied by tremendous media coverage, thus indicating the really great interest the public has in the effortless, painless way to overeat yet lose weight—starch blockers. The voodoo preparation is a protein prepared from raw soybeans and is supposed to interfere with the action of the enzyme in the small intestine that digests starch, thus the name starch blocker. Presumably much of the starch is therefore not digested, is eliminated in the stools, and thus we get fewer calories from the many starch containing foods we eat—bread, potatoes, noodles, etc.

The starch blocker idea sounds good, but it is pure, unadulterated nonsense. In the first place all proteins, and all protein enzymes are destroyed by the acid of the stomach so the starch blocker never reaches the small intestine! Second, if the starch blocker could somehow reach the small intestine intact and block the digestion of some of the starch, the undigested starch would be fermented in the large intestine, and considerable gas would be formed, with accompanying abdominal distress. Starch blockers may be effortless to take but they sure wouldn't be painless!

We wrote to the individual who presumably devised this voodoo pill, a Dr. J. John Marshall of the University of Notre Dame, to try and elicit some information, but after two months we have had no reply (and the letter did not come back).

In this case, fortunately, the FDA was promptly on the ball. They have threatened regulatory action because they consider starch blockers "drugs, not foods." Almost "overnight," the FDA claims there were 263 starch blocker manufacturers and distributors. An FDA spokesman said the agency "has received an increasing number of adverse reaction reports associated with starch blockers, including some requiring emergency room hospitalization."

How gullible much of the public is, how much many people would like to continue to stuff themselves yet take a pill and see the fat roll off, and how many others there are who would be happy to make a fast buck.

The only way we know to get fewer calories from starch is to eat less starch!

Prescription diet pills are another story entirely. During the past few decades, a few physicians who weren't too terribly concerned with ethics were quick to recognize a lucrative area when they saw one. Rather than help their overweight patients with diet control, these "fat-doctors" instead freely dispensed diet pills to suppress the appetite. The compounds and trade names vary, but most such pills contain some form of amphetamine (a stimulant for the central nervous system)—and therefore a host of possible dangers. Even the later addition of barbiturates to the pills could not completely eliminate the problems of nervousness and, sometimes, paranoid delusions and hallucinations. Other side effects often include insomnia, nausea, vascular and gastrointestinal disturbances, and hypertension. Dr. Hilde Bruch of Baylor University reports in her book, *Eating Disorders,* having treated a number of cases of psychosis caused by indiscriminate use of diet pills.

In addition, tolerance levels are quickly built up against all amphetamines. For some unexplainable reason, after about six or eight weeks the pills are no longer effective as an appetite suppressant, but what has occurred in the meantime, to a greater or lesser extent, is the development of drug dependency. To prolong the effectiveness of diet pills, other ingredients are sometimes added, including thyroid hormone, digitalis (a heart stimulant), and diuretics to promote rapid water loss. All of these substances spell trouble! The FDA has warned all physicians not to use amphetamines for weight reduction.

In *The Thin Game,* Edwin Bayrd relates the story of a young woman from Boston who managed to lose more than fifty pounds on her diet-pill regimen (composed of thirteen pills a day). Sadly, after discontinuing the pills she not only regained the entire fifty pounds, but an additional twenty as well. Bayrd calls this "tragic testimony to the net effect of any diet that does not insist on a fundamental restructuring of existing eating habits and sound nutritional reeducation."

SURGICAL ''DIETS''

Surgical weight-loss methods are too drastic and performed too infrequently to be generally considered a form of actual quackery. One procedure is jaw wiring, which allows the patient to consume only liquids through a straw. This technique carries with it the hazardous possibility of inhaling sputum or vomitus into the lungs, and contributes to tooth decay and gum disease, as well as causing the teeth to shift position.

Even more extreme is the operation known as the jejunoileal bypass. A portion of the intestine is clamped off, preventing proper absorption of food, and hence of calories. The procedure is employed only on patients who are so obese that their lives are already in severe jeopardy, since in addition to its carrying a high risk of infection and other complications, a small percent do not survive the surgery.

More bizarre still is a technique known as staplepuncture, a variation on acupuncture. The theory here is that there are "appetite-suppressing nerves" running from the stomach to the ear. When special metal clips are implanted into the ears, the dieter supposedly has only to wiggle the clips when he feels hungry and his stomach will think it has been fed. Beyond serving as a reminder not to eat too much, staplepuncture has been shown to have only one medical effect: It causes ear infections. (As we have already seen, Dr. Passwater has dispensed with that risk by proposing that the ears need only to be stroked in the right spot with the fingers.)

One surgical procedure that does show some promise in certain individuals is to staple off a portion of the stomach. This makes the stomach smaller, unable to hold so much food. Thus, one cannot eat so much. If one tries to overeat, vomiting usually results.

How to Lose Weight Safely

Fad diets often appear to be successful—temporarily. One good reason for this is that, for most people, novelty is a highly motivating factor in almost every aspect of life. Something new or different is usually appealing enough to firm up an otherwise shaky willpower, at least for a little while. Further, as we have pointed out, a number of the fad diets rely on the principle of quick water loss. The scale may indicate a lower number, but no real fat has been lost in those first few days. In any case—we don't mean to keep nagging—if there is no change in basic eating habits, the pounds are sure to reappear when the diet is terminated.

THE STARE/WHELAN DIET GUIDELINES
Sometimes we call this the "Half Diet Plus Twice," which translates roughly to eating half as much as you normally do and exercising twice as much. (That doesn't mean you can calculate the latter as two times zero.)

If you are a woman who needs to lose weight, a good diet plan should include about 1,200–1,400 calories per day, carefully selected from the Basic Four Food Groups. Most men will need closer to 1,600 calories. But for either sex, the ideal intake will depend somewhat on how active you are and on how much, and how quickly, you wish to lose. Remember that a daily reduction of 500 calories will rid you of one pound a week. (A pound of fat equals 3,500 calories.) The same result will be obtained if you decrease your daily calorie intake by 300 calories and increase your daily calorie expenditure by 200 calories—or any combination of decreased calorie intake and increased calorie expenditure that adds up to 500 calories.

We have broadened the Stare/Whelan Diet Guidelines into the Stare/Whelan Health Regimen of "Half Plus Twice Plus Nil." The "nil" refers to cigarette smoking, and you know why.

Remember that adult calorie needs decline *sharply* with age, and that there is a great deal of variability in the caloric needs of different individuals, depending largely on physical activity of the "huffing and puffing" type. *Your* recommended calorie intake is the amount that maintains your Desirable Weight, without gain or loss.

The Basic Four Food Groups will be discussed more thoroughly in chapter 11, but briefly, here is what we're talking about: the *meat group,* including poultry, fish, eggs; and dried beans, peas, and nuts (about three to four ounces total each day); the *milk group,* including all milk products (two servings a day for adults); *fruits and vegetables* (four servings a day, including one rich in vitamin C and one in vitamin A); and *breads and cereals,* whole grain or enriched (four servings a day). A "serving" does not mean a giant-sized portion; it means an average or smaller amount if you are going to keep within the necessary calorie range (and especially if you wish to include wine or a cocktail). The exception is the fruit and vegetable group, most of which are comparatively low in calories because they are mostly water. These servings can be large. A wide variety in food selection is your best assurance of providing all the necessary nutrients in sufficient amounts. The most important point to remember is to eat *less* and exercise more. In order to lose weight, you must burn up more calories than you eat.

HOW TO CHOOSE A DIET FOR YOU

Most people resist a diet completely outlined for any length of time by someone else. But others feel the need for more structure, at least in the beginning, or until they become comfortably accustomed to putting together the day's meals in such a way as to encompass the Basic Four without an inordinate number of calories.

Our first suggestion is that you check with your physician, *especially* if you have more than a few pounds to lose, in which case you should have a thorough examination before you begin. Most doctors can provide you with a basic reducing outline.

Many doctors will, and more should, refer you to a dietitian or nutritionist. You may want to request such a referral. But be cautious! Look for the principles we mentioned above (as well as those discussed elsewhere in this book). Some physicians adhere to their own pet theories, which are little better than (or occasionally identical to) those advocated by the fad diets.

If you choose to follow a regimen encountered elsewhere (in a magazine, for instance), look for one that is basically well balanced, with a minimum of gimmickry. For example, if a diet advocates beginning each meal with a piece of fruit to supposedly curb the appetite, *and it's nutritionally balanced,* it is perfectly acceptable. But really, the body doesn't care whether it receives fruit at the beginning or the end of a meal. The order doesn't matter in terms of how your body utilizes the nutrients.

Another alternative is to participate in a diet group. Those discussed below have basic low-calorie diets that are generally considered nutritionally adequate. There may be others where this is not the case, so be certain to check them out thoroughly before you begin forking over your money. (Check with your state or local health department or medical society.) Some groups will allow you to attend a free meeting or two before you join.

The effectiveness of these organizations, however, is variable, depending largely on the local leader. It is known that nonprofit self-help groups have relatively high attrition rates, and that those for commercial weight-reducing programs are even greater. The weight losses of those who do continue are generally modest. And there is no evidence that even these weight losses are maintained any more effectively than those resulting from other measures.

DIET ORGANIZATIONS

If you prefer company while you're dieting, you may find one of these diet groups helpful.

Weight Watchers has had more than 13 million registered members since its inception. It conducts meetings that involve about 550,000 people a week in the United States and is also located in several foreign countries. The total program, including the food-plan outlines, is continually updated in accordance with the latest medical findings and technologic research. In addition to well-balanced diets and behavior modification, the organization has recently added an exercise plan (allowed only after approval by each member's personal physician). Called Pepstep, it relies heavily on simple activities like walking and climbing stairs, and—like all of the Weight Watchers programs—can easily be incorporated into each person's individual life-style. Every member must weigh in at the start of each meeting. Weight changes are announced, and members are acclaimed for their losses. The classes, however, are usually conducted by nonprofessional leaders. Weight Watchers charges an initial registration fee, plus an additional fee for each weekly meeting; both are modest.

In mid-1979, *The Diet Workshop* switched from its earlier belief that dieters required a wide range of choices to the concept that what they really prefer is rigidity. Consequently, the group adopted a six-cycle diet, the first three of which are designed to be followed for only one week each. The regimen is well balanced, even though Cycle 1 includes only 750 calories a day. Since this new version is intended primarily for women, Diet Workshop suggests it be modified for male dieters (partly by cutting back on some of the cholesterol-rich items). The Diet Workshop was perhaps the first of the major organizations to include exercise in its program, and it has now added behavior modification as well. Fees are usually about $8.00 for the initial meeting and a newsletter subscription, and $3.50 per week thereafter. There are also bargain rates for those who sign up for a period of weeks.

TOPS stands for Take Off Pounds Sensibly. (Its maintenance program is KOPS: Keep Off Pounds Sensibly.) This is the oldest (1952) and largest of the nonprofit diet organizations, having several thousand members in the United States and several other countries. All the chapters are heavy on group therapy and require some medical supervision of each member. The organization is involved in nutrition research and helps support the Obesity and Metabolic Research Program at the Medical College of the University of Wisconsin in Milwaukee. But lest such endeavors sound too serious a note, we hasten to point out that TOPS is a highly social organization. After the weekly weighing-in, activities may include a speaker, skits, contests, games, and/or singing. Women's and men's meetings are usually conducted separately, however, since TOPS feels that the two sexes don't really understand each other's weight problems, anyway. The cost is reasonable, but they also welcome contributions.

Overeaters Anonymous, as you might guess, is patterned after Alcoholics Anonymous. The organization emphasizes behavior control as a means of losing weight. Only skeleton dietary guidelines are provided, the staff expecting each member to consult his or her personal physician for details. The 4,000 groups in 16 countries attest to its presumed effectiveness. There are no dues or fees; the only requirement is a sincere desire to eliminate compulsive eating.

Other groups may be less effective and/or less safe, but more expensive. *Diet Center, Inc.,* for instance, conducts a 12-week program at $20 to $25 per week, using a 750-calorie diet that is completely devoid of dairy products. This is a perfect example of the kind of diet organization that should send you speeding in the opposite direction.

QUICK TIPS FOR LOSING WEIGHT

- Counting calories is a nuisance, but an inexpensive calorie counter is useful for acquainting you with the general calorie content of most of the foods you eat. You will probably be surprised to discover that some items are much higher in calories than you had supposed—but (good news!) some are also much lower. The best calorie counter of all, however, is your bathroom scale, used weekly, not daily. Measures of weight changes should not be made daily for two reasons. First, water weight can vary from one day to the next, independent of any fat loss. Second, most bathroom scales are not sensitive enough to measure less than half-pound intervals, and weight loss per day will be less than this amount.

- Make a list of *everything* you usually eat for several days. That includes "tasting" as you cook, cleaning up the kids' plates after dinner, and the piece of candy you may have snatched (perhaps half-consciously) on your way past the coffee table. Many overweights who claim they "hardly eat anything" are startled at just how much they actually do consume. It's easy to forget about those extra 200 calories worth of casserole that were just too good to throw out. What this also does is to increase your awareness of the many times you stuff something into your mouth without even thinking about it at all. (Probably you weren't even hungry!)
- Keep between-meal tempters relatively inaccessible. An out-of-reach cupboard helps.
- Substitute low-calorie foods for regular foods as often as possible. Health-food faddists would argue that all these "diet" foods, like lower-calorie soft drinks and salad dressings, are full of "chemicals." However, there really is *no* danger associated with these foods, while there *is* often a difficulty in avoiding their higher-calorie counterparts. "Diet" substitutes can help to alleviate that difficulty. We agree that some diet products just don't "taste right," but it is usually not difficult to become accustomed to low-fat milk, diet salad dressings, low-calorie soft drinks, and so forth. Be sure the foods you buy are really low-calorie, though. Read the labels and compare. New labeling laws have made this distinction far easier for consumers than it used to be.
- Keep fried foods to a minimum, at least until you are able to see some concrete results from your weight-losing project.

When you do fry, see that foods are drained as thoroughly as possible.

- Take small bites and eat slowly. You should be able to fool your stomach into thinking you've put more into it than you really have.
- Remember two simple—but effective—table exercises. One is a vigorous shaking of the head from side to side when seconds are passed around. The other is a firm push away from the table before that fancy dessert becomes too tempting.
- Don't forget the more traditional varieties of physical exercise. That doesn't mean you have to strain the budget by joining the local country club or health center. A great number of activities like walking, jogging, jumping rope, and toe-touching exercises don't cost anything at all (although you should have a pair of good running shoes if you do much of that).
- For rounding out meals or for snacking, you may have generous amounts of "free" foods in the form of raw vegetables. Celery, green peppers, cucumbers, and all of the green leafy types contain practically no calories at all—but lots of vitamins, minerals, and fiber. (Tomatoes and a number of other vegetables are also very low in calories.) A cup of instant bouillon is a refreshing appetizer or pick-me-up at only 6–10 extra calories, but don't have it too often if you tend to have high blood pressure, because most brands are rather high in salt content.

THE NEW YOU: A SUMMARY

Fulfilling the requirements of the Basic Four Food Groups in the amounts we have recommended will take care of all your nutritional needs, and a daily calorie intake of 1,200–1,400 (perhaps 1,600 for a male) is adequate to provide flexibility in your choice of foods. We further recommend the greatest possible variety in food selection, within the scope of availability and your own food preferences. A wide variety ensures sufficient amounts of all the nutrients.

Variety and balance, on a daily basis, are the safest route to a new you—and the simplest means of keeping you that way! Finally, people should eat less to live longer to eat more. What a great slogan that would be for a supermarket chain—"We want you to buy all of your food from us, but don't buy too much, because we want you to live longer so you will be with us longer to buy more!"

CHAPTER 4

Diet and Heart Disease: Is There a Link?

BEFORE WE GIVE OUR SUMMARY RECOMMEN-dations we should report the good news that mortality (not incidence) from coronary heart disease has decreased about 30 percent in the last thirty years. This decline has accelerated so much that over 60 percent of it has occurred in the decade between 1970 and 1980. There are probably many reasons for this including improved and earlier treatment for hypertension, better coronary care in hospitals, improved training of paramedics and the public, less smoking by adult males, more exercise by more people, and dietary changes that have helped lower blood cholesterol in those individuals who have some of the known risk factors.

The Tenuous Link

In early 1980, a report called "Toward Healthful Diets" was published by the Food and Nutrition Board of the National Academy of Sciences. The National Academy of Sciences is an independent institution, not a government agency, and is highly respected in the scientific community. The Food and Nutrition Board is a special body within the academy, composed of highly qualified nutrition scientists. Among other things, the board determines the Recommended Dietary Allowances for nutrients, which are the basis for a great deal of nutrition planning in the United States.

"Toward Healthful Diets" included some controversial statements, and received enormous public and media attention. Much of the unprecedented publicity given to this report, by government agencies and industries that have promoted "low cholesterol" products, focused on the allegation that the board was comprised of scientists whose industry connections and consultancies rendered the report "biased." We thoroughly disagree with this allegation and its implications, and will address the whole topic of the science-industry relationship in a later chapter.

"Toward Healthful Diets," which, among other things, reported that there was no reason for the average healthy American to restrict consumption of saturated fat and cholesterol, led many Americans to conclude that there was little consensus in the scientific community about the relationship between nutrition and health. Actually, however, there is little disagreement about the scientific data on the subject. Instead, the controversy surrounds the nature of the *advice* to be derived from the research to date. Different scientists look at the same basic research and come to different conclusions about what it means in terms of recommending what Americans should eat.

The "diet-heart" story is an interesting, but somewhat frustrating, one. First, our bottom line: We agree with the conclusions of the Food and Nutrition Board. Other than recommending weight control, we feel it is premature to suggest basic and specific nutrient changes in the diet of healthy Americans. There is no reason to believe that normal consumption of eggs, meat, and dairy products, as part of a balanced, varied diet, poses any hazard to healthy members of the general population.

Individuals with any of the risk factors for coronary heart disease should follow the advice of their physicians.

EVOLUTION OF A MISCONCEPTION

In 1965, the American Heart Association (AHA) interpreted the extensive research to suggest that consumption of animal fats might be related to the development of heart disease and therefore advised people to change their eating habits *if* they had some of the "risk factors," particularly an elevated level of cholesterol in the blood. The recommendations were reaffirmed five years later by the Intersociety Commission for Heart Disease Resources, and in 1973 they were again restated and further elaborated upon by the AHA. At that time, the AHA advised people with elevated blood cholesterol and other risk factors not to consume more than 300 mg of cholesterol per day (a medium egg contains about 250 mg) and suggested that saturated fats be reduced by about half, from 18 percent of total calories to 9 or 10 percent, and that polysaturated fat intake should be increased from 3 or 4 percent of total calories to about 10 percent of all calories.

Up to this point, reduction of saturated fats and cholesterol in the diet was suggested for those people with elevated cholesterol and other known risk factors in heart disease. And most experts would agree that this recommendation is necessary.

However, in 1977, the Senate Select Committee on Nutrition and Human Needs, chaired by Senator George McGovern, established its dietary goals. And incorporated in the goals was the AHA recommendation to reduce saturated fat and cholesterol in the diet. The difference was that the recommendation was made for *all* Americans, not only for those at risk for heart disease. What the committee failed to recognize was that its recommendation could be backed only by early studies on the subject. There seemed to be no apparent attempt either to review more recent research results or to secure the opinions of other experts in the field. When the Surgeon General's report, *Healthy People,* was issued in 1979, followed by the HEW and USDA *Dietary*

Guidelines for Americans in early 1980, both clung tenaciously to the AHA advice, again applying it to *all* Americans.

Meanwhile, back on the industrial ranch, food processors were immersed in the development of literally hundreds of new products: low-cholesterol/fat-free/no-animal-fat/high-in-polyunsaturates kinds of products. In all likelihood a visiting alien would have quickly concluded that corn, soy, and safflower oils were some sort of magical heart protectors. We were told to use margarine instead of butter; vegetable oils instead of animal or other saturated fats; egg substitutes (like "Egg Beaters") in place of the kind that come in shells; "breakfast links" in place of sausage; and other soy products in place of almost everything else. Labeling laws had to be amended and expanded; the word "imitation" took on new shades of meaning.

The new foods—at least some of them—have been undeniably useful to many people. Gourmets may have deemed them unpalatable, but most of us found a few items to enjoy while we smugly but hopefully believed we were doing wonderful things to improve the health of our hearts. We do not deny that there is a relationship between dietary fat and cholesterol and heart disease in some of us who are at risk (those of us with elevated serum cholesterol levels). And, indirectly, a number of us were probably doing something to improve our health when we began to cut down on fat and cholesterol. Less "real" fat meant fewer calories, which in turn contributed to weight control—an indirect factor in heart-disease prevention. For many unfortunate persons, however, this wonderful theory of preventing heart disease by regulating cholesterol and fat intake grew out of proportion until it boomeranged. While many were content to coast along with less beef and a deprivation of eggs, they tended to give less and less heed to other risk factors that had already been definitely linked with heart disease: Smokers went on lighting cigarettes; the inactive remained sedentary; the obese remained overweight; individuals with diabetes or hypertension neglected the measures necessary to control these conditions. A vast segment of the public fell prey to the delusion that controlling cholesterol and saturated fat was the most important factor in eliminating heart disease.

Some segments of the food industry were only too willing to support these ideas. After millions had been invested in new product development, logic required that public anxiety be maintained at a level where the products practically sold themselves.

The coupling of diet with heart disease was a natural for the health-food industry. One of the heaviest promotions focused on lecithin, that wonder ingredient that the health-foodists alleged would "dissolve" cholesterol. (No legitimate scientific studies support that allegation in any way.) The fact of the matter is that lecithin and cholesterol combine in the body to form cholesterol ester, the compound that is considered responsible for much of the cholesterol in plasma lipoprotein (the carrier of cholesterol in the bloodstream). But the food faddists didn't limit themselves to the issue of cholesterol and fats. The door had been opened; the public was ready to try any combination of food and supplements that purported either to cure or prevent heart disease. Old folk remedies were dredged up, dusted off, and offered as the latest recipes for heart health. Descriptions ranged all the way from "revolutionary" to "what our forefathers have known for centuries."

We already know that the health-food industry pays little heed to scientific evidence. But whether the traditional food industry remained essentially unaware of the changing research results of the 1980 National Academy of Sciences study (which found that healthy people need not worry about their fat and cholesterol intake) or whether it simply chose to ignore it in favor of what the AHA was saying is a moot question. The fact is that the industry stayed with the AHA advice.

The tie-ins between the McGovern Committee and other areas of government, some segments of the food industry, the American Heart Association, and the scientific experts in this field have culminated in a hot political issue. On the one hand, the American public is still being told to change its diet. For instance, the

Consumer Nutrition Institute (CNI) has supported the recommendation for lowering dietary fat because of the results of a recent Norwegian study. A January 1982 *CNI Weekly Report* said that the study suggested that men who cut down on fat and cholesterol can reduce the chance of a heart attack. What they and others failed to recognize was that the study pertained only to high-risk coronary patients. It did *not* draw any conclusions about healthy Americans who are not at high risk for coronary heart disease.

On the other hand, more and more scientific authorities, such as the Food and Nutrition Board of the National Academy of Sciences, are trying to get across the idea that for many people major changes in the diet can very well do more harm than good; and that until more evidence is uncovered, we need to pay greater attention to those risk factors that have already been demonstrated to be causally related to heart disease.

THE POLITICS OF CHOLESTEROL

The political heat generated by the diet-heart disease controversy has been tremendous. At the present time there is unprecedented interest in this country in all facets of nutrition, and heart disease is our number-one killer. With so many agencies, scientists, and segments of industry concerned about this issue, it is not surprising that various viewpoints boil over from time to time in the form of extreme political statements.

The political reaction to the Food and Nutrition Board's report, "Toward Healthful Diets," was intense. The vested interests within the food industry and in a number of agencies (which have been advocating low-fat diets for years) took precedence over scientific criticism. Some food industries criticized the report possibly because of investment in developing low-cholesterol products, or in advertising their products as such. A number of consumer agencies would not change from a position which they had advocated for many years. Very few who attacked this report bothered to study its recent scientific findings.

The criticism that arose within the federal government was

particularly disturbing. Congressman Henry Waxman, chairman of a house subcommittee on health and the environment, called the report "startling and dangerously misleading," and said that it "threatens to set back twenty years of gains we have made in the prevention of heart disease." Dr. Wayne Calloway, executive secretary of the Nutrition Coordinating Committee of the Department of Health and Human Services, said that "although the Food and Nutrition Board says the report was written to clear up public confusion, it will probably contribute to it."

Other criticisms of "Toward Healthful Diets," and defenses of the government's Dietary Guidelines, which promoted a different viewpoint came from Carol Tucker Foreman, then Assistant Secretary of Agriculture for food and consumer services, and from Michael McGinnis, Health and Human Services Deputy Assistant Secretary for health.

But by far the strongest opponent of the report was Congressman Frederick Richmond of New York, chairman of a house subcommittee on domestic marketing, consumer relations, and nutrition. He criticized the board on numerous grounds and conducted subcommittee hearings to investigate it. His criticism may well have been a smoke screen to divert public attention from his own political and personal problems. Nothing ever came of his investigation of the board.

None of these people seemed to appreciate that the report was a scientific document. It was not a statement of government policy; the National Academy of Sciences, which is not a government agency, cannot make such statements. It was not a plot to undermine the government's health efforts or a deliberate effort to confuse the public. The report was simply an interpretation of a body of scientific evidence by a qualified, independent group of scientists.

THE STRONG POSITION OF THE AMERICAN HEART ASSOCIATION

Scientists today are in almost unanimous agreement that a great many Americans can benefit by a reduction in total calories

115

consumed *for reasons of weight control.* Obesity is indirectly related to heart disease and many other types of ill health, and, as we saw in the last chapter, excessive fat intake, because it provides 9 calories per gram versus 4 per gram of protein and carbohydrate, is the quickest route to obesity. What many scientific authorities object to are the weak assumptions on which the American Heart Association bases its recommendations about lowering fat and cholesterol intake. Briefly, these assumptions are:

(1) *That the risk of developing heart disease is primarily in proportion to the amount of cholesterol and saturated fats consumed.* True, these two substances do influence the level of cholesterol in the blood, particularly in the individual who is overweight, and elevated blood cholesterol is one of the risk factors of heart disease; but it is only one factor. The evidence shows that one's chances of having an increased level of blood cholesterol, without any other risk factors being present are very slim.

(2) *That the risk of heart disease increases directly with the level of cholesterol in the blood.* This statement assumes that *all* levels of cholesterol are related to risk; yet the actual data dispute that assumption. Application of figures from the National Cooperative Pooling Project, a study in depth conducted by the American Heart Association itself in 1978, reveals no significant difference in the incidence of coronary heart disease among persons whose average serum cholesterol levels remain below 260 mg.*

(3) *That serum cholesterol level can be controlled by limiting dietary cholesterol.* This has been shown in some studies; yet others reveal that individuals utilize dietary cholesterol differently from one another, just as they do all other substances. There are certain individuals who can eat a lot of cholesterol-containing foods and still show low serum cholesterol counts. Others eat very small amounts of these

* Raymond Reiser, Ph.D., "The Three Weak Links in the Diet-Heart Disease Connection," *Nutrition Today,* July/August 1979. Table, p. 26, calculated by J. Cornfield.

foods and still show high cholesterol counts. Furthermore, cholesterol is produced in the human body; if intake levels are low, the body tends to produce more of its own.

(4) *That by reducing serum cholesterol levels, risk of heart disease is reduced.* However, studies have not demonstrated this to be so.

(5) *That the AHA dietary recommendations, if not proven to be helpful to heart health, cannot do any harm.* However, there are indications that such dietary changes might increase the risk for a number of health disorders. A substantial increase in polyunsaturated fats can increase the requirements for vitamins A and E, and sometimes B_{12}. Polyunsaturated fats, unlike saturated fats, are oxidized in the body and can lead to liver damage and cell destruction. In one study at the Mayo Clinic, women with breast cancer had excessive polyunsaturates in their breast tissue.

REACTIONS OF THE SCIENTIFIC COMMUNITY
Medical and nutrition experts have begun to realize that the advice of the American Heart Association is not necessarily valid for the majority of healthy Americans. At best, their advice is premature. Here is what some of the experts are saying:

- Sir John McMichael, one of the world's most eminent authorities in the field of diet and heart disease, wrote in the October 1979 issue of the *American Heart Journal:*

  An immense effort has been devoted to the reduction of cholesterol levels in the blood by diet, and by drugs, and it must now be concluded that these efforts have had no detectable influence on the course of development of coronary heart disease.... Nevertheless there is a continuing flow of propaganda from epidemiologists, governments, and commercial organizations promoting a dietetic change from natural saturated animal fats to polyunsaturated fats. These represent a quite unwarranted extension of hope over experience.

- Dr. Peter N. Herbert, Head of the Section of Lipoprotein Structure, Molecular Disease Branch of the National Heart,

Lung, and Blood Institute of the National Institutes of Health, recently presented testimony on his studies to the Federal Trade Commission and later wrote: "The study has been completed, and the results in the testimony extended. We were left with little doubt that dietary cholesterol does not have a profound effect on the blood cholesterol."

- Other spokesmen from the National Institutes of Health note that by itself the diet-heart disease association presents what is an "intriguing link but not convincing."

- Dr. George Mann, professor of medicine at Vanderbilt University, voicing a somewhat more extreme viewpoint in a 1978 *New England Journal of Medicine* article entitled "Diet-Heart: End of an Era," wrote that there is little evidence to support modification of dietary intake in accordance with the current hypothesis.

- Dr. Raymond Reiser, professor emeritus in the Department of Biochemistry and Biophysics at Texas A&M University, concluded in *Nutrition Today* (July/August 1979) that "the advice the American Heart Association and others have given the public is based upon assumptions that are unsound" and that, "For three out of four persons, diet doesn't increase the risk of having coronary heart disease. Even for the remainder, cholesterol-rich and fatty foods may not be as important as we've been led to believe."

Background Basics

To assist readers in drawing their own conclusions, herewith some brief background on heart disease: what it is, what the risk factors are, what the research has told us and what it has *not* told us, and what we still need to learn.

WHAT EXACTLY IS HEART DISEASE?

Cardiovascular disease is actually a group of diseases involving the heart (cardio) and the blood vessels (vascular). Collectively, these diseases comprise the leading cause of death in the United States, claiming the lives of approximately 900,000 Americans each year. Of these, about two-thirds are victims of the specific cardiovascular disease known as coronary heart disease, or CHD.

To fully understand what coronary heart disease is, it is first necessary to understand the meaning of atherosclerosis. Atherosclerosis is an irregular thickening of arterial blood vessels created by the buildup of fatty deposits on the inner walls of the arteries. As the fatty buildup—known as plaque—continues, the blood vessels gradually become narrowed and normal flow of blood is restricted. When atherosclerosis occurs in the arteries that supply blood to the heart muscle, it is known as coronary atherosclerosis.

As coronary atherosclerosis becomes more severe, the result is coronary heart disease. The reduced blood supply to the heart may prevent that all-important muscle from being adequately nourished, from maintaining its regular rhythm, or from beating with sufficient strength to function effectively. In extreme cases, the plaque buildup may in itself result in total blockage. More commonly, the reduced blood supply tends to promote clot formation in the vessels. Even a tiny clot in an already narrowed artery can cause a heart attack. (A similar clot in the brain could cause a stroke.)

Even if the CHD victim is fortunate enough to escape or survive a heart attack, the interrupted flow of blood through the heart results in the injury or death of some of its cells, causing scarring and impairing the heart's ability to function normally. And this in turn further increases the risk of heart stoppage. This spiraling effect of coronary heart disease creates an ever-present danger. Obviously, sufferers need to be constantly aware of the various risk factors involved. But it is equally important for *everyone* to be familiar with the associated risk factors in order to reduce the chances of developing CHD at some time in the future.

WHAT ARE THE RISK FACTORS?

The precise cause—or causes—of atherosclerosis are not known. The condition usually progresses insidiously for many years before symptoms develop. It therefore becomes difficult to relate cause and effect with any degree of certainty. Coronary atherosclerosis is, however, by no means a product of "modern" living. Investigation of Egyptian mummies has uncovered evidence of the disease, and in the fifteenth century Leonardo da Vinci noted that a man was only "as old as his arteries," a concept that is still relevant today.

In 1913, a Russian scientist, Nikolai Antischokow, fed huge amounts of dietary cholesterol to rabbits and found that they developed arterial lesions similar to atherosclerotic lesions in man. Since then, a number of studies have revealed various factors associated with atherosclerosis, and several theories attempt to explain the development of plaque. Among the latter are: repeated injury to the inner walls of the arteries; transformation of the cells normally lining the arteries into benign tumor cells; virus infections; and infiltration of the inner arterial walls by fatty compounds in the blood.

During the last three decades, the popular notion developed that diet plays a key role in some way. Countless people, ourselves included, began worrying about the cholesterol and fats we were consuming. But at present, as we have stated, extensive review of the scientific and popular literature on the subject discloses that the "diet theory" *by itself*—except insofar as it relates to reaching and then maintaining Desirable Weight—is still just a theory.

Before examining dietary habits as a possible causative factor in CHD, it is first necessary to take a look at other factors that have been *absolutely* associated with the onset of atherosclerosis and heart disease. The interrelationships are considerable; in most persons, where one factor exists, so do at least one or two others.

In one category we have the so-called noncontrollable factors: heredity, age, and sex. Chances of developing CHD are greater for those with a family history of the disease, where it was diagnosed prior to fifty-five to sixty years of age. Additionally, risk increases with age and is greater for men than for premenopausal women.

In the other category are factors which can be controlled, at least to some extent. They include cigarette smoking, high blood pressure, blood cholesterol level, lack of exercise, diabetes, obesity, and perhaps stress.

Cigarette Smoking.   Autopsies have shown that cigarette smokers are at far greater risk of developing atherosclerosis than are nonsmokers, and that smokers develop the condition much more severely. This is one area where you definitely can't get away with saying, "Well, it's too late now." Smokers who quit show a decreasing risk of CHD, even after as brief a period as a few months. Eventually, an ex-smoker's chance of heart attack is no more than that of a nonsmoker. Recent studies indicate that similar hazards may result from "second-hand" smoke; that is, inhaling air containing smoke from those who are smoking.

High blood pressure.   Not only is high blood pressure, or hypertension, a serious disease in itself, but it tends to speed up the process of atherosclerosis, although the reason for this is not clear. Further, studies show that the higher the blood pressure, the greater the likelihood of a heart attack. The common type of hypertension, essential hypertension, can usually be treated with drugs, weight reduction, and possibly a sodium-restricted diet. But a major problem here, still under investigation, is whether reducing blood pressure that has been elevated for a period of time will also reduce the risk of heart attack. High blood pressure, even only a mild elevation, should not be ignored and should be treated promptly. Since there is a direct correlation between blood pressure level and risk of heart attack, at the very least a hypertensive person should attempt to prevent his blood pressure from rising further and, if possible, reduce it. (Even simply keeping the salt shaker off the dining table may be helpful.)

*   *   *

Lack of exercise. Evidence indicates that people who lead sedentary lives have a greater chance of suffering heart attacks than those who get regular exercise, either at work or at play. Some controversy still exists on this issue, most of it centering on the type of exercise that is most beneficial and the extent to which it should be practiced. Some scientists believe that moderate exercise for a period of one hour three or four times a week is beneficial. Others feel that for best heart health more strenuous exercise is required—for example, one half-hour three times a week of running or jogging. We believe that the most convincing evidence supports the idea of moderate exercise for a period of forty-five to sixty minutes, three or four times a week, as most beneficial.

However, if you decide to begin a strenuous exercise program and have led a relatively inactive life for many years, a thorough medical checkup is in order. And as your physician will advise you, start *slowly.* Don't try too much during your first few exercise periods.

Stress. It is unlikely that stress by itself can bring about a heart attack, although some evidence suggests that CHD is more likely to strike the type of individual who is aggressive, impatient, competitive, fast-paced, and constantly under pressure. Since stress is peculiar to each individual and difficult to measure, possibly it is some factor related to stress (such as cigarette smoking or hypertension) rather than stress itself that is the major culprit. Stress is a natural part of every person's life and, therefore, an important area for further behavioral research.

Obesity. The middle-aged, overweight person is two to three times more susceptible to coronary heart disease and most other diseases than a person of the same age who maintains Desirable Weight. Obesity does not actually *cause* coronary heart disease, but it aggravates and contributes to other factors that do, specifically hypertension and diabetes. Studies have consistently associated both of these risk factors with obesity. It is also found that blood cholesterol levels usually decrease with loss of weight. Weight control, therefore, becomes imperative for both the prevention and treatment of CHD.

Diabetes. Similarly, diabetes does not automatically lead to heart disease, but it is unquestionably a strong risk factor. CHD is significantly more frequent and tends to appear at an earlier age among diabetics than among nondiabetics. Proper management of diabetes, then, is also important in reducing the chances of heart attack. The most important component of treatment for the type of diabetes that begins in adulthood is getting weight down and keeping it down.

Cholesterol. As we have stated, there is little evidence that any single factor is solely responsible for atherosclerosis and coronary heart disease. While people with high levels of cholesterol (above 260 mg) in their blood have a greater chance of suffering a heart attack than those with lower levels, it is unlikely that cholesterol alone is the triggering agent. The relationship between cholesterol and CHD is not a simple one.

Cholesterol is a waxy substance found in animal foods and also manufactured by the human body. The body of a person on a completely cholesterol-free diet would still produce about one to two grams (1,000 to 2,000 mg) of cholesterol each day. The substance does not deserve the ill repute into which it has fallen during the past ten or fifteen years; rather, it is essential to human life. Cholesterol is required for many complex bodily functions, including the synthesis of the hormones responsible for both male and female secondary sex characteristics.

Fats. The association between cholesterol and fats is confusing to many people.

Saturated fats—found in meat, whole milk dairy products, coconut and palm oils, and less so in poultry and fish—have the ability to raise the cholesterol level in the blood by serving as the starting material from which cholesterol can be absorbed in the body.

123

Polyunsaturated fats are solely of vegetable origin (corn, soya, sunflower, safflower, cottonseed, and other oils) and tend to *lower* blood cholesterol *when they replace some of the saturated fats.*

Monounsaturated fats (which predominate in olive and peanut oils) also tend to lower blood cholesterol *when they replace* saturated fats, but less so than do the polyunsaturated types.

Like cholesterol, fats are not the fiends many people have been led to believe. They do have many favorable attributes. Saturated fats are found in meats and eggs, which also provide our best sources of dietary zinc and iron, and are excellent protein sources as well. Eliminating these foods from our diet may make it more difficult to meet the body's requirements for these nutrients. Fats move more slowly through the stomach than most other foods, and therefore they contribute to the feeling of satisfaction (satiety) after a meal. They also provide energy, the essential fatty acid known as lineolic acid, insulation of the body and padding for protection of the vital organs; and they serve as a transport system for the four fat-soluble vitamins (A, D, E, and K). In addition, they improve the taste of many of the foods we eat.

Lipoproteins.   Cholesterol is not soluble in water. Consequently, it must be transported through the bloodstream by means of lipoproteins, compounds made up of fats (lipids) and protein. Lipoproteins are of different types, named according to their relative weight in proportion to their volume; that is, by their density. High-density lipoproteins (HDL) have a *lower* ratio of fat to protein, as compared to low-density lipoproteins (LDL). Each kind of lipoprotein appears to function differently in relation to CHD. While the details have not yet been fully researched, some evidence points to the possibility that LDL may be associated with *increased* risk of CHD and HDL with *decreased* risk. In some manner HDL may "lure" cholesterol away from the arterial walls and carry it to the liver, where it is metabolized and destroyed.

It is known that as people approach maturity their concentrations of HDL are lowered, and those of LDL raised. Theoretically, that fact might account for the increased risk of heart disease with advancing age. Marathon runners, known to be at low risk of atherosclerosis, have higher levels of HDL. According to a newly completed study by the Cardiac Rehabilitation Division of Methodist Hospital in Houston, even more modest runners and joggers tend also to gradually raise their HDL levels over a period of time. Thus, we have another "plus" for moderate, frequent exercise. Additional studies of heart-disease victims of every age, race, and sex have shown lower levels of HDL and increased levels of LDL. However, the full implications of the relative amounts of high- and low-density lipoproteins in the blood currently remain unclear.

Combined factors. Any combination of the risk factors discussed above will act to further increase the possibility of heart attack or coronary atherosclerosis. At worst, the risk can be increased more than ten times that of someone who is not subject to any of the risk factors. Of the controllable risk factors, the combination of hypertension, cigarette smoking, and an elevated blood cholesterol is the most hazardous.

WHY DID DIET BECOME SUSPECT?

Undoubtedly, the effectiveness of certain kinds of nutrients in the prevention and treatment of certain disorders—for example, vitamin C in the prevention of scurvy and iodide in the prevention of goiter—led scientists to seek out nutritional causes and cures for coronary heart disease.

With a view toward uncovering clues to a link between diet and heart disease, U.S. Army pathologists examined the hearts of some 300 American soldiers killed in the Korean War. The average age of the soldiers was just over twenty-two; all were in apparent good health at the time of death, and none had shown previous signs of CHD. Yet the coronary arteries of more than three-fourths of them clearly revealed early signs of atherosclerosis. Over 15 percent had at least one artery narrowed by 50 percent or more; 3 percent had an artery completely blocked. In contrast, young Japanese men studied by the same doctors displayed much less arterial narrowing or thickening of over 50 percent.

The researchers suggested that the presence of atherosclerosis in otherwise healthy Americans of such a young age might implicate diet as a causative factor. Further, the fact that the arterial thickening and narrowing among American soldiers was considerably more severe than it was among the Japanese, whose diet is relatively low in fat, tended to put the blame on dietary fats. To lend additional support to this theory, other scientists noted that during the past fifteen years the heart-disease rate in Japan has tripled—ostensibly as a result of a national shift toward a more Westernized (higher-fat) diet. On the other hand, the environments in which Japanese and American soldiers were raised differ in many respects other than diet. And Westernization reflects many changes in addition to diet.

Chemical analysis of atherosclerosis deposits have revealed high contents of fats and cholesterol, but whether the deposits occur because those substances are present in the blood in excessive amounts, or whether they would simply occur anyway, is still a matter of debate. Investigation of CHD in countries around the world has failed to uncover any clear evidence of diet as the sole contributing factor. In some countries CHD and heart attacks are virtually unknown, while in others (like the United States) they are a leading cause of death. Since dietary practices vary from country to country, researchers have sought to analyze the differences in relation to CHD. So far, the results have tallied up to a big question mark.

Studies of Diet and Heart Disease

Heart attack is statistically associated with high levels of blood cholesterol. We know that this correlation exists. What we do not know is whether the relationship is one of cause and effect. Many elderly people with high blood cholesterol have never suffered a heart attack, while others with low blood cholesterol are dying of

CHD. Further, in the presence of other risk factors, it has not been established that merely reducing the blood cholesterol level will prevent a heart attack.

ANIMAL STUDIES

Animal experiments have shed some light on a diet-heart disease association. The most that such studies have contributed, however, is to substantiate that a possible relationship does exist. And even that much must be interpreted with caution, since the animals' dietary requirements and utilization of nutrients are often vastly different from man's.

EPIDEMIOLOGIC STUDIES

Epidemiology is the study of the distribution of disease and associated factors in human populations. Evidence derived from this type of study is useful in assessing human risk. However, epidemiologic investigations into the diet-heart disease association have reported conflicting results, even though they utilized very similar techniques. We mention here only two of many such studies.

The 1970 International Cooperative Study, which analyzed records of some 12,000 men from seven countries over a ten-year span, is the largest study conducted to date. Dr. Ancel Keys, the principal investigator, found that men who ate the greatest amount of saturated fats had the highest rate of new cases of CHD.

However, another large study, the aforementioned "Pooling Project," reported no association between diet and heart disease. This study, which combined the records of several smaller analyses into a single population of 7,000 men, found no evidence of a greater number of CHD cases among those who consumed diets high in saturated fat.

METABOLIC TESTS

Metabolic nutritional tests are closely monitored human experiments that study the way foods affect the chemical levels and energy balance of the body. Studies have demonstrated that an increased consumption of saturated fatty acids produces a corresponding increase in blood cholesterol levels, and, conversely, that decreased consumption of saturated fats accompanied by a corresponding increase in unsaturated fats, particularly polyunsaturated fats, results in lower blood cholesterol.

Unlike the findings related to fatty acids, studies measuring the effects of dietary cholesterol intake have produced conflicting results. Some have shown a direct relationship between the amount of dietary cholesterol and blood cholesterol levels, while others have not.

CLINICAL TRIALS

Clinical trials are studies in which human volunteers agree to modify their diets and to submit to careful medical evaluation for a period of time. An ideal study of this type—one that would answer the question, "Can a change in diet prevent heart attacks?"—would have to be carried out over a long period of time on many subjects and could easily cost upwards of $1 billion. The prohibitive cost necessarily means that these investigations are less than ideal; but despite their limitations, some clinical trials have made important contributions.

First, these studies have shown that it is possible to modify the food habits of individuals without an unacceptable change in nutrient intake. Second, they have shown that dietary changes that reduce consumption of saturated fats and cholesterol, and that increase polyunsaturated fats, do lower levels of blood cholesterol. Third, they have *not* shown that these dietary changes *by themselves* reduce the development of coronary heart disease. You will remember, however, that there are multiple risk factors for CHD and that the interaction between them requires further study. Thus, it is possible that diet may indirectly influence other risk factors.

WHAT WE HAVE LEARNED

The results of one study may indicate a correlation between diet and heart disease; the next study is just as likely to show none at all. Even the most extensive, long term, carefully controlled studies in the United States have failed to produce clearcut evidence of dietary causes of heart disease. But research has provided us with a substantial amount of information about the CHD/diet association. These data can be summarized as follows:

- Persons living in industrialized societies have more heart disease and higher average blood cholesterol than persons in less developed areas.
- People suffering from CHD generally lead less active lives and have higher levels of total blood cholesterol.
- Individual differences in blood cholesterol levels occur in persons with the same dietary habits.
- Dietary changes can lead to reduced blood cholesterol for some, but not all, people.
- Consistently high blood cholesterol levels increase the risk of developing CHD, *when other risk factors are also present.*
- Atherosclerosis is the result of many factors; among them are both genetic and environmental factors.

Should the American Diet Be Changed? Three Schools of Thought

While new information is sought, different scientists interpret the evidence in different ways.

''CHANGE NOW''

Some independent scientists and many associated with organizations such as the American Heart Association maintain that there is sufficient evidence right now to warrant substantial changes in the American diet *for the entire population.* They recommend general decreases in consumption of total calories, total saturated fats and cholesterol; and a general increase in the proportion of unsaturated fats (particularly polyunsaturated fats).

These groups base their recommendations for immediate changes on two assumptions: First, that it is only a question of time before a direct connection between these dietary factors and CHD is verified. They believe that if resources were available to conduct a proper study, the findings might be conclusive. Second, they argue that these dietary changes can only benefit the general public and would have little or no possibility of adverse effects. They note that in the past other successful public-health efforts have been based on equally limited or incomplete information.

"WAIT FOR CONCLUSIVE EVIDENCE"

Representing a somewhat different point of view are those who point to the current failure to verify a direct relationship between the risk of CHD and diet alone. Some scientists argue that since such a link has not been firmly established, it would be premature to recommend changes in the American diet. Others go a step further; they do not accept the assumption that reducing total calories, dietary saturated fats and cholesterol, and increasing polyunsaturated fats would have no adverse effects.

Not all public-health-policy recommendations based on limited and indirect evidence have been successful. One example is the now disproven link between excessive weight gain and increased risk of toxemia during pregnancy. At one time, pregnant women were frequently advised to limit weight gain to only twelve to fifteen pounds in order to minimize the risk of toxemia. Newer studies, however, demonstrate that such weight restrictions not only do not prevent toxemia, but contribute to cases of premature birth and other complications in pregnancy. Currently, a gain in weight during pregnancy on the order of twenty to twenty-five pounds is generally recommended.

A particularly extreme viewpoint is offered by David Reuben, M.D., in his preposterous *Everything You Always Wanted to Know About Nutrition*. Based on the results of one rabbit study and one human study, he concludes: "The final result is absolutely undeniable. Here it is, once and for all: Changing the fat content of your diet will not decrease the risk of heart attack," and, "If you don't want to get sick, you better eat cholesterol." That kind of nonsense is blatantly inaccurate.

Most legitimate scientists, however, are somewhat more conservative in their opinions. Those opposed to broad dietary modification for the general public, except for the reduction of total caloric intake in order to reach and maintain Desirable Weight, note that further study of other possible dietary factors is needed. They contend that unless the causes of CHD are more firmly established, changes in diet are not indicated for the healthy individual.

INDIVIDUAL PRESCRIPTION

A third, more moderate group has concluded that although there is some evidence to suggest a relationship between diet and CHD, the risks do not apply to everyone. This school of thought advocates individual assessment and therapy based on an analysis of all suspected risk factors, both voluntary and involuntary. These scientists believe that multiple risk interpretations for the individual patient are superior to a campaign designed only to modify the diet of every American—again, we emphasize—except for reaching and then maintaining Desirable Weight. To our way of thinking, this is by far the most sensible approach.

GOING TO EXTREMES: THE PRITIKIN DIET

Many nutritionists would agree that the average American diet is too rich in fat. But Nathan Pritikin, director of the Longevity Research Institute in Santa Barbara, California, true to the nature of all good extremists, has carried that idea a step further. As co-author of the book, *Live Longer Now,* and later as author of the best-sellers, *The Pritikin Program for Diet and Exercise* and *The Pritikin Permanent Weight Loss Manual,* he has advocated a diet almost totally devoid of fat. On the Pritikin diet, fat provides less than 10 percent of total calorie intake, as compared to the 40 percent generally consumed today and the 30–35 percent recommended by proponents of the "change now" school of thought, such as the American Heart Association. (The weight-loss version of the Pritikin diet is simply a lower-calorie version of the original.)

Mr. Pritikin is not a doctor and is totally lacking in professional credentials in nutrition or medicine. After Mr. Pritikin himself suffered a heart attack, he decided to engage in self-guided research. But his lack of training in the areas of nutrition and medicine did not deter him from making extraordinary claims for his diet program. An almost fat-free menu, Pritikin contends, will not only prevent heart disease but will even *cure* it. This would be a remarkable contribution to medical science, if only it were true. (Mr. Pritikin, like many authors of fad-diet books, has expanded the virtues of his diet beyond its original realm. His latest book now claims that the diet is useful in the prevention and/or treatment of constipation; cancer; disturbances of the liver, gallbladder, and kidney; gout; osteoporosis; premature aging; headaches; blood-clotting disturbances; hypoglycemia; diabetes; and high blood pressure, as well as heart disease. But the claims about heart disease are still the diet's main "selling point.")

As you certainly realize by now, heart disease involves a great many risk factors, of which diet is only one possibility. Many Americans, particularly those who need to lose weight, could benefit from a moderate cutback in high-calorie, high-fat foods. But reducing fat intake to practically nothing severely limits the choice of foods. Most good sources of protein and calcium are not permitted on such a diet, so very careful dietary planning is needed to prevent deficiencies of these nutrients. Also, a very low-fat regimen tends to leave the dieter feeling continually hungry. It is difficult to adhere to such a diet plan for very long.

The Pritikin diet, unlike some fad diets, isn't medically dangerous, at least in the short term. However, it quickly becomes intolerable, especially when you realize that the regimen cannot live up to Pritikin's remarkable promises.

WHAT ABOUT SALT?

You have probably heard that sodium, and substances containing it such as table salt (chemically, sodium chloride), are also bad news when it comes to heart disease. The problem with sodium is that it may contribute to the development of high blood pressure in susceptible individuals. As was mentioned before, hypertension is not only a significant disease in itself, it is also a risk factor for coronary heart disease. Patients who have hypertension are often treated with moderately sodium-restricted diets, in addition to appropriate medication.

Some health authorities have also suggested that the general public should cut down on sodium. Many surveys have shown that Americans consume far more sodium than needed. Physicians are also aware that many people have mildly elevated blood pressure and don't know it, since it often produces no symptoms. Quite a few people who regard themselves as healthy really do suffer some degree of hypertension.

So the federal government, in its Dietary Guidelines for Americans, and other health organizations have recommended that we all cut down on salt. Unlike fats and cholesterol, sodium occurs mostly as part of a condiment, salt. You can cut down on it simply by decreasing the use of salt in cooking and keeping the salt shaker off the dinner table.

But we should warn you that, like many other things in nutrition, the now-popular advice to cut back on salt is controversial. All the current furor over salt in the American diet may give the impression that scientists agree on how salt (or more correctly, its sodium component) affects our health. This is not the case. The subject is surprisingly complex, and medical experts disagree vigorously over whether healthy individuals should decrease dietary sodium in order to reduce their risk of hypertension.

Right now, the bottom line is this: Cutting back on salt won't hurt you. Although our bodies require sodium, the amount needed is small, and you would have to make very extreme changes in your diet to make yourself sodium-deficient. Many scientists think that decreasing dietary sodium will reduce our risk of hypertension. The evidence for this, however, is not conclusive. Whether or not to cut back on salt is a matter of individual choice. It may indeed turn out to be beneficial to your health. *But there are no guarantees.*

Dietary Factors That Have Never Been Shown to Affect Heart Disease

Inevitably, the search for answers has given rise to all manner of nutritional nonsense surrounding CHD. Based on legitimate research, we know that dietary cholesterol *may* be causally related to heart disease—and we also know that certain other dietary factors have never been shown to have *any* causative association. The alleged "studies" that are sometimes quoted to back up these useless claims are at best haphazard, ill-conceived, and uncontrolled; at worst, they are nonexistent.

SUGAR

The flurry created some years ago by Dr. John Yudkin, who proposed that sugar caused heart disease, continues to attract a crowd. We will discuss his illogical theory more thoroughly in chapter 7 on sugar. The fact is that Yudkin's conclusion was based on studies involving only a few subjects; the hypothesis was not borne out by other research.

LECITHIN

Earlier we referred to the health-food mongers' contention that lecithin is capable of dissolving both plaque and cholesterol. Some of the organic wags insist that fertilized eggs contain more lecithin than others and thus "neutralize" the cholesterol in their yolks. (That's the same cholesterol we're not sure we even have to worry about in the first place.) The theory is not very appealing; it is not supported by good evidence, and we remind you that lecithin is produced in the human body and is found in many foods other than eggs. We do not need supplements of it.

ONIONS AND GARLIC

The alleged healing properties of these two related foods have their roots in early folklore. At one time or another, garlic and onions have been viewed as cure-alls for almost everything, but heart disease continues to crop up as a favorite point of attention. Onions, garlic, and some other members of that aromatic family contribute a great deal to the tastiness of many dishes, but that is the extent of their magic.

OTHER ''WONDER PRODUCTS''

Even if we could take them seriously, there is no way that space will allow a discussion here of the plethora of foods, dietary supplements, and other products that promise—or have promised or will promise—to protect against heart disease. We hereby dismiss them all on a single general note: If a true wonder cure does arrive on the nutrition scene, the medical profession will have no wish to keep it a secret.

Summary Recommendations

In general, diet and health are strongly related. While evidence does suggest that there may be a relationship between nutrition and coronary heart disease, the specifics are still elusive. If you have other risk factors for coronary heart disease, or if the condition has already been diagnosed, you and your physician will have to decide what, if any, dietary changes are appropriate for you—especially if you have an elevated blood cholesterol level. Today most physicians consider a cholesterol level of 260 mg/100 ml, or above, as elevated, and some regard anything above 220 mg/100 ml as elevated. Certainly, if your cholesterol is 200 mg/100 ml or lower, changes in diet are not necessary or advisable.

The best nutritional advice for persons who are *not* suffering from symptoms of coronary heart disease and who *do not* have some of the "risk" factors is to eat moderate amounts of a variety of foods. A diet that includes foods from each of the Basic Four Groups is your best "nutritional insurance." Variety minimizes the possibility of excesses and maximizes the likelihood of obtaining all necessary nutrients.

The principle of food variety also applies to fats and oils, and encompasses animal fats as well as those from vegetable sources. In moderation you may include all types of meats, cheeses, milks, and other dairy products that tempt your palate and meet your budget. But do note those key words, *in moderation.* All fats and oils, from whatever source, are high in calories, and all contain the same number of calories per gram. If weight control is a problem, as it is for many, you will need to avoid excessive amounts, not only of fats but also of alcohol, another potent source of calories. Throughout the week, alternate meats with relatively lower-fat poultry and fish. Meats and fried foods should be thoroughly drained before serving. Beer and wine have far fewer calories than the same amount of a cocktail or highball.

Far more knowledge of the relationship between diet and heart disease will be needed before other specific recommendations can be advanced for the healthy individual. The decades of research have been arduous and frustrating. Often after years of effort a study has produced results that shed practically no additional light at all on what was already known. We still have much to learn, but while progress has been slow, it has also been steady. Until more evidence is in, there is no justification for normally healthy individuals of Desirable Weight to worry about eating meat—or eggs—or butter. A balanced, varied diet is still the best aid to good health.

Until more is learned about the role of diet in heart disease, we need to place greater emphasis on *known* risk factors: cigarette smoking, hypertension, obesity, and underlying conditions such as diabetes.

CHAPTER 5

The "Poisons" in Our Food

AMERICA HAS BEEN SWEPT BY A WAVE OF chemical phobia. Distortion of facts about the safety and quality of the national food supply has paved the way for a new and growing form of nutritional rip-off. Again and again, the public is bombarded with the misinformation that "organic" food is better than "regular," and that "natural" everything is better than "artificial."

The Nature of Organic Food

To begin with, the term as it is generally used is a misnomer. By definition, all food and all other substances derived from living matter are organic. To insist that only some kinds of food are organic is like saying that only some kinds of water are wet. What the health-food hucksters are actually intending to promote are goods that are *organically grown;* that is, raised without benefit of commercial fertilizers and without the protection of pesticides. This organic method sometimes produces a finished product that is smaller, spottier, and worse-looking than its pesticide-grown counterpart. The contention that there is any other basic difference in the quality of the final product, however, is completely without merit.

FERTILIZER

There is just no way to change appreciably the nutritional content of any food by the way it is grown. An apple, for instance, is an apple. Because of genetic differences, the fruit from one tree may be juicier than that from another; or it may be fresher; or it may taste better because it was harvested nearer to its peak of ripeness and therefore contains more sugar. But no apple will ever contain as much vitamin C as an orange, simply because it is an apple and all apples are lower in vitamin C than all oranges. Likewise, the difference between one apple and the next is unrelated to the kind of fertilizer used. An apple tree may produce more fruit or fruit that is superior to that of another tree, sometimes because of good agricultural practices, such as adding fertilizer or protecting the fruit with pesticides.

As the battle between commercial and organic fertilizers rages on, a large segment of the population seems to have lost sight of one of the first principles of elementary botany: that plants do not utilize food in the same way that animals do. Nutrients must be in inorganic form for them to be of any use to a plant. Organic fertilizers—such as manure, compost and cover crops—have the advantage of improving the texture and workability of the soil, but the nitrogen and phosphorus in them that eventually become available to the plants must be converted to inorganic salts, just like that in commercial fertilizers. This conversion of organic compounds of nitrogen and phosphorus to inorganic compounds is made by soil bacteria.

The disadvantages of organic fertilizers are more apparent: Often plants have to wait a good while for them to be broken down into usable components, whereas the nutrients in commercial fertilizers are immediately available. If a plant doesn't have enough of these needed elements, it simply will not grow well.

Mineral nutrients, including trace elements, may or may not be present in plants in adequate amounts, depending on whether they are present in the soil. If iodine (in the form of iodine salts) is missing from the soil, there will be none in plants grown in that soil. If manure from animals fed on these plants is later used for fertilizer, the iodine is still missing and will continue to be missing until it is introduced from some other source.

Very often manure does contribute a little "something extra"—usually, it is in the form of *Salmonella,* a common culprit in "food poisoning," but other harmful organisms may be present as well.

Dr. Ruth Leverton, one of the nation's most respected nutrition educators and a former spokesperson for the USDA's Agricultural Research Service, notes: "There is no proven, substantiated basis for claiming that plants grown with only organic fertilizer have a greater nutrient content. . . . The type of fertilizer used . . . is not a determining factor in the nutritive value of the plant." Yet no amount of explaining or drawing diagrams of chemical structures will convince those who do not wish to be convinced.

PESTICIDES

The 1981 battle between California and the "medfly" again brought the topic of pesticides to the headlines and television evening news. A small group of California consumers pressured Governor Jerry Brown to withhold aerial sprayings of a very effective and very nontoxic pesticide—malathion. And the results were frightening: The entire California fruit and vegetable crop was in jeopardy until Secretary of Agriculture John Block stepped in to put an end to some very serious nonsense. Malathion was sprayed, and most of the crops were saved. But the example should linger in the minds of consumers when they hear demands to "stop the spraying."

Insects compete with people for food. Robert Rodale* and his

* Robert Rodale is publisher of *Organic Gardening* and *Prevention* magazines, both founded by his father, J. I. Rodale.

organic-gardening cult would have us believe that strong, healthy, organically fed plants are virtually immune to insect attack, that the critters devour only plants that are too weak to defend themselves. The difficulty here is that no one has informed the insects. Likewise, they seem to care little that they are expected to succumb to "natural" antibug sprays concocted from pulverized garlic, soapsuds, and red pepper; or that interplanting with members of the onion family is supposed to discourage their presence.

And insects comprise only one group of pests. For the vast array of plant diseases, and fungus and other unwanted growths, onions and garlic are about as helpful as a rain dance. A century ago, the one million people who starved to death during the Irish potato famine would have indeed appreciated a pesticide to control the fungus blight that destroyed the potatoes.

Pesticide residues are closely monitored by the federal and state governments. Such sensitive testing equipment has been developed that it can now detect parts per *trillion* of any residues. (One part per trillion has been described as a single grain of sugar in an Olympic swimming pool full of iced tea.) Acceptable standards are such that produce in grocery stores and supermarkets exhibits a higher level of safety than that grown in many backyards. Further, there exists *no documented case of illness caused by the consumption of pesticide residues on food purchased in any grocery store or supermarket.* When you occasionally see what appear to be the remains of pesticide sprays on fruits and vegetables, you can rest assured that they no longer contain harmful amounts of the active ingredients. (And we assume you wash produce before eating or cooking it, anyway.)

Regulations are strict. Pesticides cannot be used on food within a specified length of time before harvesting date (the number of days varies with the substance used). Farmers who depend on the sale of produce for their livelihood can ill afford to ignore safety laws.

Pesticides have been the subject of unwarranted attacks ever since the intense controversy over the use of DDT in the late

1960s. According to Helen Kelly, a researcher with the American Council on Science and Health, the debate over DDT was a prototype for later pesticide conflicts.

DDT certainly did not deserve its infamy. Ms. Kelly reports that this insecticide has been credited with saving one hundred million lives as a result of its use against insect-borne diseases, particularly malaria. Agricultural use of DDT, to kill insects that destroyed crops, was also very effective. DDT enjoyed a great popularity as an insecticide, partly because it combined high toxicity for insects with low toxicity for people and animals. Thousands of individuals, military and civilian, had their clothing dusted with 10 percent DDT powder while they wore it, without ill effect. No toxic effects were noted in the 130,000 people employed as DDT sprayers, or in the 600 million people who lived in repeatedly sprayed dwellings. The only documented instances of DDT poisoning in humans were the result of massive accidental (or suicidal) ingestion of the insecticide.

Nevertheless, a strong anti-DDT movement formed in the 1960s, prompted by the popularity of Rachel Carson's *Silent Spring*. Eventually, in 1972, most uses of DDT were banned in the United States, despite the fact that no real health hazards would have been caused by continued use of this insecticide.

DO YOU GET WHAT YOU PAY FOR WHEN YOU BUY ORGANIC?

Do you get what you pay for when you buy organic produce? No! Losses in the field are bound to be higher when foods are grown organically. With a lower per-acre yield, growers must inevitably jack up their prices. Retailers in turn raise prices still further, usually beyond the ordinary markup, just by virtue of the fact that the food is "organic." What happens is that the consumer ends up paying up to twice as much, or even more, for that organically grown apple that we explained earlier is essentially the same as any other apple. Well, maybe not quite the same. There's a fair chance that this one might be scabby or wormy.

(Of course, there's always the argument that the high cost is for the extra protein supplied by the worm.)

What is of greater concern than the economic rip-off is that foods sold as organically grown are not necessarily what they purport to be. Public hearings held before New York Attorney General Louis Lefkowitz in 1972 uncovered the fact that of 2,000 organic-food samples tested each year, approximately 20 percent show traces of pesticide residue, with about 1 percent having levels in excess of approved tolerances. (This does not mean that the foods were unsafe. Tolerance levels are quite strict.) More specifically, Dr. Elmer George, director of the New York State Food Laboratory, testified that of fifty-five food products labeled as being organic taken from a wide sample of metropolitan New York stores, seventeen of them contained pesticide residues. The levels were approximately the same as would be found in regular foods. But what that means is that over 30 percent of such test items as spinach, dried apricots, carrots, nuts, raisins, tea, and sesame candy was being sold as high-priced organic food, when in fact it had been treated with the same pesticides as other foods. Whether those same foods had also received commercial fertilizers could not, of course, be tested. Once the plant has absorbed its basic food components, there is no way to detect where they originated.

Naturally, exposure of the pesticide frauds was very upsetting to "legitimate" organic growers. What all this led to is a forceful movement by the health-food industry to convince the government that it must enforce the "organic" label. To put it another way, they are requesting that government certify their unfound claims.

While Robert Rodale vainly attempted to defend the wonders of organic foods during the hearings, he was questioned about his credentials for disagreeing with so many prominent authorities. His answer: "I am trained as an English major in journalism. I admit I don't have the background." Perhaps even more appalling is the "expert" advice continuously doled out to an unsuspecting public by health-food-store employees. As was also brought out at the organic hearings, staffers may have been hired off the street ten minutes earlier, but once on the floor and dealing with the consumer, Assistant Attorney General of New York State Mindell said that they "speak in terms of nutrition as if they had Ph.D.'s from Columbia and Heidelberg and sixteen other places." Vincent White, confidential investigator for the Bureau of Consumer Frauds, testified: "A few establishments told me that if you are a little heavy, and you eat organically grown food, you might lose some weight or you might be free of diabetes." It is precisely this kind of nonsense that is not only hazardous to the pocketbook, but can be hazardous to one's health as well.

OTHER EFFECTS ON THE ECONOMY

A few farmers have managed to "go organic" with a fair amount of success. But as officials of the U.S. Department of Agriculture point out, a great part of the reason they have been able to make it is because of government regulations and pest control on surrounding land. Neither a plant disease nor a horde of insects is likely to zero in on a single isolated farm.

If organic-farming methods were to be adopted as the sole means for raising plants, however, the effect on both nutritional status and worldwide economy would be nothing short of disastrous. Limited supplies and higher production costs would cause prices to skyrocket. Dr. Norman Borlaug, Nobel Prize winner for his development of new strains of wheat and other improved methods of food production, has estimated that, "If the use of pesticides in the United States were to be completely banned, crop losses would probably soar to fifty percent, and food prices would increase fourfold to fivefold."

It is precisely our new technology that is helping to relieve starvation and premature death in countries around the world. The hungry are grateful for something to eat. In a battle that pits man against the world of insects and plant diseases, the underfed do not quarrel with the use of pesticides. And most assuredly, they do not care what kind of fertilizer is used to increase yields.

Natural vs. Synthetic

The human body is no more discerning than the lowly plant about its sources of nutrients. Take the much-talked-about vitamin C, for instance. Vitamin C, or ascorbic acid, is a specific chemical compound. It is the same compound whether it is found in an ordinary orange, an organically grown orange, a vitamin capsule, or as a synthetic substance in an orange drink. Your body needs its daily supply of vitamin C, but it couldn't care less in what form it enters the mouth.

The healthmongers, of course, will tell you otherwise—and in this case they have a twofold scam going. Not only are you urged to eat only organically grown oranges, but you are advised to supplement them with "natural" vitamin pills. Vitamin C (and other) supplements ostensibly derived from natural sources generally sell for three or four times as much as other supplements, which already sell for far more than the cost of manufacturing them. Not only is there no difference whatsoever in the vitamin content, the real hoax here is that most of the time only a small amount of the vitamin is "natural"; the remainder is synthetic, just like the synthetic vitamin C in most vitamin pills.

CHEMICAL PHOBIA

While it is seemingly acceptable to include synthetic compounds in dietary *supplements,* the health foodists continue to blast away at any such compounds being added to *food.* Masses of otherwise intelligent individuals have been gripped by the unfounded fear of chemicals in their food, certain that if they cannot pronounce it, it must be harmful. In an attempt to allay some of these fears, many food processors have added to labels an explanation of the reasons for each additive contained in a given product. But the strange-sounding names continue to instill fear.

What most people fail to realize is that *all* foods are composed of chemicals. You might easily be repulsed by the offer of a hot,

144

steamy solution containing, among other things, caffeine, tannin, geraniol; and butyl, isoamyl, phenyl ethyl, hexyl and benzyl alcohols—yet what we have just described is a simple cup of tea, organically grown or otherwise. And what about those supernatural apples and oranges? Apples contain fascinating compounds like phlorizin and isoflavones; and those vitamin C-laden oranges also give us tangeretin, tyramine, synephrine, and citral. Natural grape flavoring contains at least nineteen different chemical compounds. Artificial grape flavoring contains only five, yet the public is led to believe that only the natural version is "safe." If every item in any given food market were to be labeled with a list of all the chemicals it contained, many people would apparently end up eating nothing at all.

Chemical additives, whether natural or artificial, are there for a reason: to provide the consumer with a better product at a lower price. The argument is often raised that some substances are included only to lengthen an item's shelf life. That is true, but it is necessary to carry that premise a step further with two important points: a) An item that has a longer shelf life in the store will also remain fresh for a longer period in the home; and b) a longer shelf life means lower costs to the manufacturer and the retailer, and ultimately to the consumer. As we will see a bit later, there are a great many other reasons for putting additives in foods—and they benefit the processor only insofar as they provide a more satisfactory product for the consumer.

THOSE PREADDITIVE ''GOOD OLD DAYS''?

It is difficult to find in the history books a time when additives were *not* introduced into foods. The practice dates from the time food was first used in trade and is mentioned as far back as the writings of Pliny.

During those early days, additives were used solely for the benefit of the vendor. In eighteenth-century London, bread was often mixed with chalk, alum, and bone ash, both to make it whiter and to stretch it further. Milk thickened with flour was sold as cream. Tea frequently had iron filings added to it to make it weigh more, or it was stretched with used tea leaves collected from local inns.

By the mid-nineteenth century in New York, a concoction known as "swill milk" was common: Cows were fed on the exhausted grains that had been used to make beer and whiskey, and the resulting milk was watered and then colored with chalk or plaster of Paris to disguise its thin bluish color. England had by now progressed to diluting brown sugar with potato flour or tapioca. Cocoa contained colored earth, and sulfuric acid was added to vinegar. Ochre, red lead, and other substances were used as colorings in a variety of foods.

Borax, carbolic acid, and similar compounds sometimes helped prevent further decay in food that was already partly rotted, often making it look good enough to sell. There was fake coffee and fake maple syrup. Foods of every sort were colored and adulterated to reap a greater profit by defrauding the buyer. And on top of all that, the medical field was so unsophisticated that illness could rarely be traced to contaminated food.

The advent of the Food and Drug Administration, together with advances in medical science, put an end to many of these swindles, at least in the United States. Deliberate adulteration and careless contamination continue to occur, of course, but the ceaseless efforts of the FDA and local health authorities attempt to keep such cases to a minimum. Not only foods but supplements, too, became subject to FDA regulations. For instance, Lydia Pinkham's Vegetable Compound, a "female remedy" that was well known not so many years ago, fell by the wayside when it was learned that it provided symptom relief because it was composed largely of alcohol. Likewise, the use of approved additives is carefully monitored and their safety continually tested.

ADDITIVES AREN'T ALWAYS ''UNNATURAL''

It will probably surprise many people to learn that a great many food additives are totally natural compounds. A prime example is a substance called calcium propionate, often used as a mold inhibitor in bread. It may sound like something concocted strictly in the laboratory, but it is actually a substance that is normally used and produced in the human body; and it is also found naturally in many foods such as Swiss cheese. The amount of calcium propionate in a Swiss cheese sandwich is enough to preserve two loaves of bread. What, then, would we have to gain by *not* using this "chemical"? The answer is nothing but a lot of moldy bread.

But lest calcium propionate sound too unfamiliar to you, consider the many common natural substances that are also used as food additives: mustard, pepper, yeast, citric acid (a natural component of oranges, lemons, and other citrus fruits), and coloring matter from such foods as beets. Furthermore, the three chemical compounds that account for 93 percent by weight of all food additives used in America are sugar (sucrose), corn sweeteners (corn syrup, dextrose, and fructose), and salt (sodium chloride). Nothing could be more natural than that threesome.

Fallacy: "Natural" Is Safer

Several years ago, over 100,000 turkeys in Europe died after eating moldy peanut meal. The feed was made from perfectly "natural" peanuts contaminated with the perfectly natural black mold, *Aspergillus flavus,* which produces a perfectly natural deadly substance known as aflatoxin. We now know that aflatoxin, which can form in a variety of nuts and grains, especially if they have been stored while still damp, is also one of the most potent carcinogens known to animals and man. In low doses over a period of time, it can probably cause liver cancer in humans. Careful monitoring by the Food and Drug Administration has prevented aflatoxin from becoming a major problem in the United States, but many other countries are less fortunate. The toxin is the suspected cause of death for many children in the Orient, where it is commonly found as a contaminant of moldy rice, the staple food of the region.

Another type of mold toxin caused thousands of deaths in

Russia during World War II. One year during the war, heavy fighting prevented farmers from harvesting their crops. The crops remained under the snow all winter. By spring, the food supply had run extremely short, and the over-wintered crops were desperately needed for food. Unfortunately, a toxin-producing mold had grown on the grains during the winter, and when the plants were harvested and eaten, many people were fatally poisoned.

Similarly, a parasitic fungus known as ergot attacks certain types of highly susceptible rye and wheat. The active components of this purple mold are a number of alkaloids with a basic nucleus similar to the hallucinogen LSD.

Ergot has been used medically for centuries: Because it causes muscles and blood vessels to contract, it is helpful in treating migraine headaches and at one time was used to induce abortion; but in large doses it can lead to numbness or a painful burning sensation of the extremities, even producing gangrene and violent death. The LSD-like effects, which became known as Saint Anthony's fire (because that saint had been martyred by burning), have resulted in countless deaths and serious injuries. In 1944, over 40,000 people were said to have died as a result of ingesting the mold. New evidence suggests that the events of the Salem witch trials were influenced by the fact that much of the general population had consumed contaminated rye. And as recently as 1951, there was an outbreak of "bread poisoning" in France, during which many victims tried to fly off buildings or screamed in terror that they were being surrounded by fire or attacked by prehistoric beasts. (It is only fair to mention that one hypothesis has held that mercury poisoning was also involved in the French incident.) In addition to inducing Saint Anthony's fire, the very natural ergot has also been linked with tumor formation in certain laboratory animals.

But like aflatoxin, ergot does not present a major concern in this country because the bread processors are aware of the dangers and how to guard against them, and because samples of rye and wheat products are now routinely examined by the FDA.

Although authorities continually warn, both molds *could* lead to disaster because many smaller organic growers are unaware of the problem and do not know what to watch for or how to prevent it.

SOLA DOSIS FACIT VENENUM

Or, to translate the observations of the famed Renaissance physician Paracelsus, "Only the dose makes the poison." Were that not so, the entire world population would have been wiped out long ago.

The health foodists holler about the minute traces of artificial additives put into processed foods, and a large segment of the rest of society has become frightened and taken up the cry. What they seem not to realize is that a great many—perfectly natural—foods commonly found in the American diet contain "poisons." They are not contaminants; they are a part of the inherent structure of the food itself.

Consider some of the other undesirable substances found in our natural food supply. But before you panic, keep in mind that these "poisonous chemicals," like artificial additives, are present in *extremely small amounts.* Our forefathers have been eating them long enough to testify to their safety.

- In addition to arsenic, potatoes that are partly "green" contain solanine, a poison that can cause neurologic and digestive problems, and even death when consumed in large amounts. (It is always wise to cut any green portions out of potatoes.)
- Shrimp and many other kinds of seafood contain copper and even higher amounts of arsenic than are found in potatoes.
- Lima beans contain hydrogen cyanide, as do a variety of other seeds and nuts.
- Certain kinds of peas (genus *Lathyrus*) contain substances that can cause bone and central-nervous-system toxicity.
- Almonds contain the deadly amygdalin, a cyanide-containing compound.

149

- Carrots contain carototoxin, a dangerous nerve poison; and myristicin, a hallucinogen.
- Onions have substances that interfere with the activity of the thyroid gland.
- Radishes contain two chemicals that promote goiter by interfering with iodide absorption.
- Broccoli, similarly, has five goiter-causing chemicals.
- Cabbage, brussels sprouts, turnips, and rutabagas all contain substances toxic to thyroid metabolism.
- Spinach and other plants are high in oxalates, which, among other effects, can interfere with iron absorption. Popeye would have been disturbed to learn that spinach is also suspected of having adverse effects on the gastrointestinal tracts of young children.
- Beets, spinach, and a number of other vegetables are very high in nitrate—far higher than the allowable amounts of nitrite artificially added to other foods such as bacon.
- Olives contain benzo(a)pyrene, a potent carcinogen.
- Bananas contain substances called pressor amines that tend to raise blood pressure, and which at least one study has indicated may be related to the high incidence of heart lesions in a particular group of Africans. According to Richard L. Hall in *Nutrition Today,* if just one gram of banana pulp were injected into the human body (note that this is a very common way of testing laboratory animals), the effect would be similar to that of 50,000 bee stings.
- Avocados and many cheeses also contain pressor amines.
- Oranges contain a chemical toxic to human embryos.
- Cereal grains may contain relatively high levels of selenium (a cousin of arsenic, but even more deadly) if they have been grown in soils naturally rich in that element.

The list is almost endless. But, we repeat, the levels of these toxic substances are so low that their presence in any of the foods just mentioned has never been found harmful, even if you indulge in supersize helpings. You would have to eat an entire carload of lima beans, for example, in order to consume a lethal dose of cyanide—and even the most outrageous overeater is unlikely to be that enamored of limas.

Nevertheless, the eating public is fortunate that the federal government has not seen fit to apply the Delaney Clause* to foods *without* artificial additives. A great many of them would never pass inspection. We could no longer enjoy our carrots and potatoes and avocados and apples. They would all be banned.

THE ''SAFETY'' OF NATURAL HEALTH FOODS

This is perhaps the biggest myth of all. It is doubtful that regular customers of the health-food industry have any idea they are living dangerously every time they partake of certain of their purchases.

Sassafras, for instance, has for a long time been considered a nostrum for many ailments and a health-food favorite. Until 1960, it was also used as a (natural) flavoring for root beer. At that time, experiments confirmed that one of its components, safrole, caused liver cancer in some animals, and that led to its inevitable demise as a food additive. The health-food-store explosion in the early seventies found sassafras back on the market as the key ingredient of a "health-food" tea. Eventually, the FDA again came into control. The sale of sassafras root is still allowed, but only as long as all of the safrole in it has been removed.

Apricot kernels, or aprikern, were other favorite health-food goodies. Unfortunately, they also contain hydrogen cyanide, but in considerably higher amounts than do lima beans. Not too many years ago a three-year-old girl suffered cyanide poisoning after eating approximately fifteen of the kernels.

Kelp is another favorite fad item. We have already mentioned

---

* This is the food-safety clause that specifically relates to cancer and food additives. It reads: "No additive shall be deemed to be safe if it is found to induce cancer when ingested by man or animal, or if it is found, after tests which are appropriate for the evaluation of the safety of food additives, to induce cancer in man or animal." The law will be discussed further on p. 154.

that it is often so rich in iodide compounds that it can affect the thyroid and lead to metabolic disorders. Moreover, elevated urinary arsenic levels in patients undergoing neurologic investigations were traced to the use of kelp tablets purchased as health-food supplements.

Bone meal, that wonder substance the health quacks tell us is better for our teeth than fluoride in the water, is frequently contaminated with lead. There are a number of cases on record in which regular users developed lead poisoning and/or leukemia.

Natural wild honey commands a great deal of attention these days. Few people know, however, that if the honey has been manufactured by wild bees feeding on such natural plants as azalea, rhododendron, or mountain laurel, the product can be highly poisonous.

In varying degrees, both arsenic and selenium are found *naturally* in the soil and are taken up by the plants that grow in it. Selenium, *in trace amounts,* is necessary to human nutrition, and arsenic may also be essential; but in excess amounts both are lethal. Yet selenium compounds are regularly promoted by the manufacturers and retailers of dietary supplements.

Salt (sodium chloride) is yet another very natural substance, although, except for sea salt, its sale is not restricted to health-food stores. Humans must have some small amounts of both sodium and chloride in order to survive. But we generally consume ten to twenty times more than the necessary amounts. Some persons with high blood pressure (hypertension) may benefit by limiting their salt intake. A number of cases are on record of children mistaking salt for sugar, eating it in very large amounts, and developing "salt poisoning" with vomiting, fever, respiratory distress, and sometimes convulsions and death.

Raw (unpasteurized) milk has made a recent comeback as a health-food favorite. Proponents claim to be concerned that pasteurization destroys too many nutrients in the product. We assume that their quest for natural milk overrides any fears about contracting a natural case of diphtheria, typhoid, or undulant fever.

The greatest, and perhaps most widespread, danger of health-foodery probably lies in the popular use of health-food herbs, either as smoking substances or in teas and capsules. Many preparations contain psychoactive substances; that is, compounds that produce euphoric, hallucinogenic, or marijuanalike effects. In a 1976 article on herbal intoxication, Dr. Ronald K. Siegel reported in the *Journal of the American Medical Association* that 192 different herbs were available as smoking substances, and that almost half of these preparations were psychoactive, with symptoms that sometimes persisted for days. Additionally, 396 herbs and spices were used in tea preparations, of which 43 were psychoactive. A great many of these herbs would be prescription items if sold in a pharmacy.

Some of the hallucinogenic herbs commonly used in teas are: nutmeg (which, along with carrots, parsley, and other items, contains the hallucinogenic agent, myristicin), catnip, periwinkle, thorn apple, and mandrake. Other substances are used variously as stimulants, tranquilizers, sedatives, analgesics, or euphoriants. Health-food manufacturers are happy to make available lists of the wonder claims of an array of their herb/spice products. Were you gullible enough to believe the propaganda, it would take only a quick glance to assure you that the right combination of herbs and spices could cure or prevent virtually anything that ails you. Magic, indeed! One can't help conjuring up visions of bubbling caldrons and cackling ladies in long black gowns and tall peaked hats.

But if you substitute common sense for gullibility, it should be no surprise that all euphoria and tranquilizing and stimulation and hallucinating might at least make you *think* you feel a bit better—for a little while. Of course, if you don't feel better, or even if you do, ultimately you may very well feel a whole lot worse. But it's your money—you might as well get *some* reaction from it.

THE DELANEY CLAUSE

"No additive shall be deemed to be safe if it is found to induce cancer when ingested by man or animal, or if it is found, after tests which are appropriate for the evaluation of the safety of food additives, to induce cancer in man or animal."

That brief paragraph, which was added to the 1958 Food Additives Amendment by New York Congressman James J. Delaney, has since created more controversy about food safety than any other single piece of legislation. Because no one seems able to agree on what is meant by "tests which are appropriate," the survival of every food additive hangs in balance, even those that have been used safely for decades.

But while the Delaney Clause was admirable in intent, it did not—and does not—take into account the technological advances of the past twenty-plus years. The original idea held that there was no threshold level for cancer; that is, that there was no level below which the amount of a possibly carcinogenic substance could be considered safe. That assumption constitutes what is known as *zero tolerance*. At the time the Delaney Clause became law, testing equipment could not detect levels lower than fifty parts per million. Thus, that figure was accepted as "zero," simply because scientists could not detect anything below that level.

Today, however, testing equipment has been developed that is sensitive enough to find one part per *billion* (the equivalent of one inch in sixteen thousand miles); some substances can be detected in amounts of one part per trillion. Nonetheless, the clause still reads "in any amount." Thus, the zero-tolerance-requirement level has fallen from fifty parts per million to one part in a billion or trillion. Clearly, benefits must be considered as well as risks. As HHS Secretary Richard S. Schweiker has stated, the clause should be redefined in "terms of risk-benefit ratio."

Toxicity, as we have seen, is a question of amount. If one consumes enough of anything, it can be lethal. Even water can be toxic, and that applies whether we are speaking of the chlorinated, fluoridated variety, or the all-natural, "unadulterated" type from spring-fed wells.

And while too much of any substance can be harmful, the converse is also true: *There is no substance so toxic that small amounts of it cannot be used safely.* To put it another way, there is for every substance a level below which it can be used safely. Of course, there is the argument of how that level is to be determined, since it varies for each substance. Common sense and research studies together should provide fairly accurate bases for judging. Take nitrates, for instance. The amounts found naturally in many common vegetables, as well as in human saliva, are a great deal higher than the legal limitations allowed when nitrate (or nitrite) is used as a food additive—yet the issue of whether to ban added nitrate (or nitrite) entirely has been the subject of a good deal of controversy.

Nowhere in the Delaney Clause is there any mention of weighing benefit against risk. Thus, America is presumably expected to ignore the fact that the nitrite added to bacon, hot dogs, and other foods prevents growth of the deadly botulism organism, *Clostridium botulinum.* What the clause focuses on, instead, is that nitrate in the human stomach is converted to nitrites, and then to those carcinogenic nitrosamines. That the nitrosamine levels are negligible—even lower than the trace amounts formed from human saliva and consumption of nitrate-containing vegetables—is given no weight by strict Delaney adherents.

The Delaney Dilemma forcefully commanded widespread public attention in 1969 when four laboratory rats developed bladder tumors after receiving huge doses of a three-substance mixture that included cyclamates. (Saccharin was another of the three.) For some reason, cyclamate was singled out as the sole culprit, and the Department of Health, Education and Welfare proposed a limit on its use. That wasn't enough for certain public-interest groups, however. Ultimately, congressional pressure forced a total ban on the substance, forcing hundreds of thousands of persons to do without a popular noncaloric sweetener that had made it easier to fight the battle of the bulge, and that was also very useful and convenient for diabetics. The scientist who had conducted the original studies subsequently protested that his findings had been misused, with the result that a great deal of additional research has since been conducted—to the tune of several millions of dollars. Today it seems conclusive that cyclamates as they were used were not and are not human carcinogens. Unfortunately, they are still prohibited in the United States, but available in Europe and other parts of the world.

Practically everyone knows that penicillin and other antibiotics can be lifesaving in small doses. At higher dosage they can be toxic, even death-dealing. Just as no one is likely to consume a carload of those cyanide-containing lima beans at one sitting, neither is one likely to knowingly ingest a pound and a half or so of penicillin in a short period of time. The problem is that the Delaney Clause leaves no room for applying even the most minute amount of logic.

THE DELANEY CONTROVERSY

Few pieces of food-related legislation are as controversial as the Delaney Clause. It has been hailed by some as the "last backstop" of consumer protection and condemned by others as based on "poor science." When researchers from the American Council on Science and Health asked individuals who were very involved in discussions of the clause whether they thought that it had outlived its usefulness, they obtained a wide variety of responses.

Dr. Arthur Upton, former director of the National Cancer Institute, maintained that "the authors of the Delaney Clause recognized [the] limitations [in our knowledge of risks and benefits] and determined that the safest and most effective strategy to protect human health was to ban the addition of known carcinogens to the food supply insofar as possible." In Dr. Upton's opinion, "that rationale remains equally sound today."

Conversely, Dr. J. M. Coon, professor of pharmacology at Jefferson Medical College in Philadelphia, said, "The Delaney Clause is not necessary or desirable to protect the consumer from the addition of carcinogenic chemicals to foods. The Food, Drug and Cosmetic Act provides the authority, without the Delaney Clause, under which the FDA can restrict the use of any food additive which it judges has not been proved to be safe. Any food additive can be ruled unsafe under the provisions of the act that apply to 'adulterated foods.' "

Ellen Haas of the Community Nutrition Institute, a Washington-based public-interest group, replied this way when asked if the clause had outlived its usefulness: "Just the opposite. The Delaney Clause continues to provide consumers with critically needed protection against chemicals deliberately added to food. . . . The economic, social, and psychological consequences of human cancer are too grave to permit or allow cancer-causing risks that are unnecessary."

Peter Barton Hutt, former chief counsel for the FDA, told the American Council, "For the past fifteen years, I have steadfastly adhered to the view that the Delaney Clause is a trivial statutory provision that is not worthy of serious public discussion. It adds nothing whatever to general safety provisions that have existed in the law for over seventy years. . . . The Delaney Clause never was intended, and in fact is not, a statement of scientific principles. It was, and remains, a statement of public policy. . . . The real issue is what represents the most rational public policy [in light of our uncertainties about the scientific principles]."

Finally, Murray D. Sayer, assistant general counsel of the General Foods Corporation, warned, "In our zeal to attain the unattainable, 'zero risk,' we may well be committing future generations to a critical food 'crunch.' . . . The Delaney Clause, as it has been implemented into a 'no-risk' philosophy, no longer represents a rational food-safety policy and should be amended."

PROPOSALS FOR CHANGE

Though many proposals have been made to modify the Delaney Clause (and the entire Food, Drug and Cosmetic Act of which the clause is a part), they all generally fit into one of three categories: those that seek to delete the clause; those that seek to include risk-benefit analysis in the regulatory process for food additives found to be cancer-causing; and those that seek to include a certain amount of risk assessment in the regulatory process (without, at least explicitly, weighing the risks against the benefits). Many bills proposing these changes have been submitted to the House and Senate for consideration.

In the House, Representative Thomas S. Foley of the state of Washington has introduced a bill which would delete the Delaney Clause. This bill would remove the special emphasis placed on cancer and animal testing, thus making the regulation of food additives subject to the more general safety provisions of the Food, Drug and Cosmetic Act.

Representative James Martin of North Carolina has introduced a bill that would allow evaluation of both the risks and the benefits of food additives.

Representative Clarence J. Brown of Ohio has introduced a bill that would retain the Delaney Clause but would give the FDA several regulatory options in dealing with additives that were shown to cause cancer in animal tests, if those additives were not scientifically determined to present a substantial risk to human health. This bill would also allow the benefits of the additives to be taken into consideration.

In the Senate, Senator Orrin Hatch of Utah has introduced a bill that would make comprehensive changes in the whole Food, Drug and Cosmetic Act. Among other things, the Hatch bill proposes to modify the Delaney Clause so as to require that the FDA undertake a thorough risk assessment (i.e., determining the extent of risk) before banning food additives found to be carcinogenic.

The Food Safety Council has also proposed a comprehensive revision of food-safety laws that would probably remove the Delaney Clause. Under the council's system, a special technique called a "decision tree" would be applied to the estimation of all risks presented by food additives. Cancer would not be singled out as a special risk. Rather, it would be treated in the same way as other significant health hazards.

5: *The "Poisons" in Our Food*

CLEAN OUT THE POISONS!

Chemical phobia has left the public wide open to the foolish notion that they must keep their collective digestive system free from poisons. The theory that all diseases are caused by putrefaction of food in the intestines has been around for at least a century. Over the years, people have been advised to conduct regular clean-out campaigns with the use of bran, tonics, enemas, abstinence from certain foods, or periodic total fasting.

More recently, the health-food stores have come to the rescue with concoctions designed to function as internal cleansers. The general recommendation is that they be ingested regularly, either instead of or in addition to other "natural wonder" foods. One health-foodist (an ex-airline stewardess with no nutritional training whatsoever) advises a swig of lemon juice and distilled water every thirty minutes throughout the day.

The ideas behind all this are nothing short of sheer nonsense. The human body is a marvel of biologic engineering. One of its built-in safety features is a digestive system specifically designed to rid itself of toxic wastes. Under normal health conditions, a balanced diet and regular meals will handle the job nicely without additional outside help. Furthermore, repeated use of any kind of laxative can interfere with normal metabolism and lead to unnecessary dependency.

Artificial Additives

The American diet today contains approximately 3,000 different food additives, counting both the natural and the artificial. Excluding the "big three"—sugar, corn sweeteners, and salt—that make up 93 percent by weight of all additives, the average American consumes slightly less than 10 pounds of food additives during a year's time. And of those 2,997 other additives, a mere 30 account for about 80 percent of that 10 pounds.

Ten pounds of artificial and natural additives may sound like

159

either a little or a lot, depending on your viewpoint. You need to keep that figure in perspective. The average American also consumes an average of 119 pounds of potatoes in a year and, in so doing, ingests about 9,700 milligrams of toxic solanine. That's enough to do in a horse *if* it were to be taken in a single dose.

WHY DO WE NEED ALL THOSE ADDITIVES?

We don't actually "need" them, in the sense that our bodies can function perfectly well without them. But some of the additives consciously placed in foods unquestionably provide us with a food supply that is more plentiful, economical, attractive, healthful, and altogether more enjoyable than we would have without them.

Let's take a brief look at a few common additives and what they do:

Antioxidants, such as BHA and BHT, are used to prevent the browning of processed fruits and to prevent fat rancidity in vegetable shortenings and oils, or in foods containing those substances.

Other preservatives, such as sodium benzoate and calcium propionate, are used to control growth of molds in baked goods, cheese, and fruit juices, among other foods.

Emulsifiers, such as mono- and di-glycerides, lecithin, polysorbate 60, propylene glycol, and monostearate, prevent separation of the ingredients in products like salad dressing, margarine, pudding and cake mixes, and chocolate.

Stabilizers and Thickeners, such as gum arabic, pectin, and carrageenan, maintain a smooth, uniform texture and provide desired thickness in such foods as ice cream, chocolate milk, salad dressing, cream cheese, jams, jellies, candies, and sauces.

pH Regulators, such as citric acid, lactic acid, and sodium bicarbonate, control the acidity or alkalinity of many food such as gelatin desserts, processed cheese, and instant soft-drink mixes.

Nutrient supplements, such as vitamin and mineral compounds, improve the nutritive value of a host of foods.

Flavoring agents, including both natural and synthetic flavors such as lemon, garlic, and all variety of herbs and spices, are used to improve the flavor of many foods regardless of season.

Coloring agents, including both natural and synthetic substances like carotene, caramel color, beet powder, and artificial colors, are used in numerous foods to enhance their appearance.

Miscellaneous additives include a number of different kinds of substances. Some prevent caking and foaming; others are used for firming and bleaching. The group also includes flavor enhancers such as MSG (monosodium glutamate) and nonnutritive sweeteners like saccharin.

Without food additives, salt would stick in the shaker during humid weather; peanut butter would separate; many canned and frozen fruits and vegetables would be mushy; ice cream would be crunchy with ice crystals; and many foods would spoil in a short period of time.

SACCHARIN

We have already explained the need for administering high test doses of a suspected carcinogen if it is to elicit an effect in experimental animals. Nevertheless, there is a point beyond which the dose is so high that it poisons the animals' normal metabolism.

In the case of saccharin, the one experiment that confirmed a causative relationship to cancer was, to put it mildly, overzealous. Pregnant rats, and then their offspring, were fed saccharin at *5 percent* of their total diets, an enormous proportion of the diet of any animal. Dr. Frederick Coulston, director of the Institute of Comparative and Human Toxicology at Albany Medical College, observed that this dose was "so high it interfered with the normal physiological state of the animals. It resulted in loss of greater than 10 percent body weight, which is usually accepted by most toxicologists to indicate a chemical dose that is too high."

While animal studies provide valuable clues to possible human health hazards, decisions should not be based on one study alone. Of the twenty animal studies performed with saccharin since 1959, only that *one* study concluded that saccharin can cause bladder cancer in animals. All other investigations yielded findings that were either ambiguous or pointed to saccharin's safety.

The saccharin case is a bit unusual in that, unlike other additives, we have accumulated a large body of data gathered from *human* studies. Widespread investigation of diabetics, who use much more saccharin than nondiabetics, has shown no adverse health effects. Similarly, studies of bladder-cancer patients have also failed to show any link between the disease and saccharin consumption. This conflict of findings points out the obvious fact that animal tests cannot be accepted automatically.

The National Academy of Sciences, in attempting to steer a middle course through the saccharin controversy, has not agreed that saccharin should be banned immediately. They argue—and rightly so—that in cases where human risk is small or unproven, individuals should have the freedom to make their own decisions.

As of this writing, the proposed FDA saccharin ban has been thwarted by congressional action—so we will continue to have this artificial sweetener with us for at least the next couple of years.

NITRITE

A continuing and rather complicated controversy surrounds the food additive, nitrite. Actually, nitrite and the closely related nitrate are not just food additives; they also occur naturally in many vegetables, are produced in our saliva, and are found in some drinking-water supplies. Both nitrate and nitrite are manufactured by the bacteria that normally reside in our intestinal tracts. Less than 5 percent of our nitrite intake comes from its use as a food additive.

Under some circumstances, nitrites can combine with naturally occurring food components called amines, to produce nitrosamines. Nitrosamines are known cancer-causing agents. Scientists are devoting a great deal of effort to reducing the amount of nitrosamines in foods, and they are also concerned about the possibility that nitrosamines might be formed in the body, after food is eaten. But this concern about nitrosamines became a secondary issue after it was suspected that nitrites themselves might cause cancer. This "suspicion" came to public attention rather abruptly.

In August 1978, the Food and Drug Administration and the Department of Agriculture announced the banning of sodium nitrite as a food additive. Nitrites and nitrates have long been used as ingredients in cured meats (and in some poultry, fish, and cheese products) for two reasons: 1) They inhibit the growth of bacteria, including those that cause botulism, a deadly form of food poisoning; and 2) they give these products their characteristic color and flavor. The agencies realized that if they banned these additives abruptly, the risk of botulism would increase. Therefore, they planned a gradual phaseout, combined with research to develop alternate methods of preventing bacterial growth in cured meats.

What prompted this action? The agencies had received results from a study, performed under contract to the FDA, indicating that nitrite had caused lymphoma, a type of cancer, in rats. Federal officials, including the then commissioner of the FDA, were convinced of the validity of the study. They publicized the alleged hazard widely and issued very definite public statements. Yet others, including the scientist who had performed the rat study, were not so sure. He believed that his findings were "only suggestive."

Questions about this scientific study arose shortly after the phaseout was announced. Eventually, an extensive review of the study was conducted for the FDA by independent scientists. After examining 50,000 slides of tissues from 2,000 rats, the independent experts found a much lower incidence of lymphoma than had originally been reported. In fact, the incidence of lymphoma was so low that there was no longer any evidence that nitrite had caused this type of cancer in rats. The reevaluation showed that a comparison group of rats *not* fed nitrite had *more* lymphomas than the test rats that *did* eat the nitrite.

In August 1980, two years after the phaseout was announced, FDA and USDA dropped all plans to ban nitrite. Unfortunately, the fears of hot dogs, bacon, and other cured meats developed by many during the two-year nitrite scare are harder to "phase out."

The nitrite incident is a good example of what can happen when the government acts too hastily on the basis of preliminary or questionable scientific data. Scientists themselves don't regard findings as reliable until other experts in the field have reviewed them thoroughly; this is called "peer review" in scientific lingo. Unfortunately, peer review is not always a part of government regulatory procedures. The case of nitrite shows why it should be.

The nitrite scare had devastating effects on the processed-meat industry. Many important products were threatened—nitrite is an ingredient in foods that make up a tenth of our total food supply. Suddenly, industry scientists were faced with an urgent need to find alternatives to nitrite, so that they could produce products that would be both bacteriologically safe and nitrite-free. This would have been an enormous research task.

Consumers were also hurt by the nitrite scare. Had nitrite been banned unnecessarily, we would have been forced to learn new ways to store and handle nitrite-free meats in order to prevent the growth of dangerous bacteria. The consumer education effort would also have been enormous.

The nitrosamine problem remains, of course, but it can be dealt with. Nitrosamines have been found in cooked bacon and, in tiny amounts, in some beers and scotch whiskeys. However, most breweries, as well as most bacon processors, have already changed their processing methods in ways that will block nitrosamine formation.

GROWTH HORMONES AND ANTIBIOTICS

Our national meat supply has come under growing criticism during recent years because of growth hormones in animal feed and the use of antibiotics to prevent animal diseases. The safety of both groups of substances is constantly checked, and neither has ever been found harmful in the amounts used. Yet controversy reigns as to whether or not they are subject to the rules of the Delaney Clause.

Diethylstilbestrol, better known as DES, is a synthetic form of estrogen used to promote rapid cattle growth with less feed and, therefore, lower cost to the consumer. The hormone came under attack a few years ago after several cases of vaginal cancer were discovered in women whose mothers took DES (prescribed to prevent miscarriage) during pregnancy.

Current regulations require that DES in beef be discontinued a full seven days before slaughter, but radioactive tracer studies may still detect minute amounts of DES in beef livers—although not in any other part of the animal. The traces are restricted to one or two parts per billion (ppb). The consumption of 25 tons of beef liver at 2 ppb would constitute a dose of only 50 mg of the estrogen DES. The facts approach the ridiculous when you also consider that not only is estrogen present in human saliva and as an important female hormone, it is also found as a natural component in eggs, carrots, soybeans, rice, oats, barley, potatoes, apples, cherries, plums, garlic, parsley—and even in those two health-giving superfoods, wheat germ and honey. And you can be sure that "natural" estrogen is indistinguishable from synthetic estrogen.

During its lifetime, a 500-pound animal that is fed DES-treated feed eats 500 pounds less total feed than an animal eating untreated feed, and it reaches a marketable weight of 1,000 pounds in 34 fewer days. If DES were to be discontinued, the estimated cost to consumers ranges between $500 million and one billion dollars annually. The hypothetical danger of consuming minuscule amounts of synthetic estrogen that might be present in just the *liver* of beef lends no justification for banning DES as a cattle-growth stimulant.

The FDA seems to seek to terrify consumers that they are at risk of cancer if they have eaten beef from DES-treated cattle. The *FDA Consumer,* the agency's official magazine, quoted Lester M. Crawford, former director of the FDA Bureau of Veterinary Medicine (BVM) as saying, "DES was long ago shown to be carcinogenic," and that Americans are "enshrouded in a number of myths," including "the myth of the dose-response curve—the idea that you'd have to eat a 'carload' of beef from DES-implanted cattle 'to get cancer.' " Nevertheless, the FDA continues to use dose-response curves for evaluating the cancer-causing potential of DES. And you *would* have to eat a "carload" of beef to consume a medically significant amount of DES.

The furor over the use of antibiotics in farm animals is similarly puzzling. The drugs are not used to treat foods, but they are extremely valuable in controlling animal diseases, some of which may also be dangerous to humans. Most antibiotics so used travel straight through animal intestines without ever getting into the meat at all. Those that do reach muscle tissue are present in only minute amounts and are destroyed during cooking.

TESTING FOOD ADDITIVES

The process for testing all new additives introduced into the American diet is very time-consuming and complicated. The battery of tests lasts from two to seven years, and each substance is studied in a variety of ways and in a variety of animals. Different animal species are necessary because most, if not all, of them utilize substances differently from man. Rats, for instance, can easily tolerate doses of vitamin A at levels that would be toxic to man. We also now know that certain varieties of rats are more susceptible to carcinogens than others.

As thoroughly and carefully as additives are tested, there is simply no way to prove 100 percent safety of any substance at every level. Throughout this chapter we have repeatedly attempted to show that toxicity is a matter of amount. There is no substance on earth that will not cause toxic reactions if the dosage is high enough—and there is no substance, however potent, that cannot be rendered safe if the dosage is low enough. Our regular food supply is often safer than products found in health-food stores.

Of course you don't want dangerous substances added to your food. Neither do we. We all need to be informed about substances that are potentially harmful in large amounts. We also need to know how to weigh benefits against risks.

Banning additives that are perfectly harmless in restricted amounts makes about as much sense as banning automobiles and electric stoves. There is a point beyond which the consumer must accept responsibility for the products he or she chooses to use.

ORGANIC, HEALTH, AND NATURAL FOODS— SOME DEFINITIONS

With so much "loose talk" about these three classes of foods, it might be helpful to have some definitions and suggestions. We know of no legal definitions for these three classes of food, not even definitions suggested by the FDA or any other government agency. However, one of us (FJS) was invited by the Department of Consumer Affairs, City of New York to give testimony and define these terms at a public hearing in December 1971.

After the testimony had been prepared, FJS thought that if his senior colleagues in Harvard's Department of Nutrition agreed, it would greatly strengthen the testimony. All of them did, and their names were appended to the testimony. It is of interest that of the nine professors who signed the testimony, four were M.D.'s and five were Ph.D.'s. This testimony was published in the summer of 1972 in the *Journal of Nutrition Education*, and as far as we know, this is still the only publication suggesting specific definitions of these three classes of food. The following remarks are from that publication:

> *Health Foods*—"All edible foods are health foods and promote physiologic or psychologic health—regardless of whether they are purchased in a neighborhood grocery store, a supermarket, or a so-called health-food store."
>
> *Organic Foods*—"All foods are organic—protein, fat, carbohydrate, and vitamins—because they are, in the definition of the chemist, organic compounds containing carbon. The organic-food enthusiasts should speak of 'organically grown foods,' by which they mean foods grown on soil fertilized with organic fertilizers—manures or composts of various types—and foods grown without the use of chemical pesticides."
>
> *Natural Foods*—"All foods are natural or are manufactured from natural foods. However, many individual nutrients—for example, most of the vitamins—may be either of natural origin or manufactured synthetically. However, these individual nutrients are not foods; they are nutrients."

The Harvard Nutrition Department's recommendations at that time (and today) are:

1. "We think regulations should be adopted that no foods be singled out as 'health foods,' because all edible foods, when properly used in a balanced diet, are conducive to physiologic or psychologic health—regardless of whether they are purchased in a so-called 'health-food store,' an ordinary grocery or supermarket, or in a special section of the latter."
2. "We think regulations should be adopted that no foods be singled out as 'organic foods,' because all foods are organic. Foods that are fertilized only with organic fertilizers, rather than manufactured chemical fertilizers, and on which no chemical pesticides have been used in the growing and no chemicals of any kind added during the processing and preparation (food additives) might be identified as 'organi-

cally grown foods.' However, even this terminology is not correct, because much of any soil is composed of inorganic substances that are necessary for the growth of plants."

3. "We think that regulations should be adopted prohibiting the use of the term 'natural foods,' because all foods are natural or are manufactured from natural foods."

Those interested in this subject should read the entire testimony (*Journal of Nutrition Education*, Summer Issue, 1972, pp. 94–97).

CHAPTER 6

Diet and Cancer:
Taking Advantage of Fear

CANCER—THE DIAGNOSIS DREADED BY PA-
tient and nonpatient alike. National surveys reveal it to be the
most feared of all diseases. And with good reason: Less is known
about the actual causes of cancer than about any other major
disease. More properly, we should say *group* of diseases, since
there are actually between 100 and 300 different kinds of
cancers,* each with its own patterns of etiology and often with
differing means of prevention and treatment. Every organ and
tissue in the body is subject to attack, a frightening prospect indeed. While great strides have been made in the treatment of
some types of cancer, we are still helpless to combat many others.

Fear provides an open invitation for quackery. It seems that
people will do almost anything to avoid the possibility of
cancer—as long as it doesn't require too much effort. A large
segment of the population finds it far easier to stamp its feet and
fuss about a purely hypothetical risk like food additives (which

* Some experts view certain cancer subgroups as variations of a single
disease, while other authorities consider every form as a separate disease.
Thus, the discrepancy in the total number of different types.

have never been shown to cause cancer in the amounts used in the human diet) than to give up cigarette smoking, which is a proven contributor to lung cancer. This witless displacement of concern simply does not jibe with scientific data.

The Cancer "Epidemic": Is There One?

Cancer in its various forms comprises the second leading cause of death in the United States. Last year approximately 395,000 Americans died of the disease, and an estimated 765,000 new cases were diagnosed.

In spite of these formidable statistics, the United States is *not* in the midst of a cancer "epidemic." The National Center for Health Statistics reports an increase in the overall cancer death rate in the past few decades: from 113 per 100,000 population in 1930, to 125 in 1950, to 132 in 1976. But this increase is by no means large and cannot support the notion of an epidemic. Further, as is readily apparent from the graphs below, the *only* form of cancer mortality that has been increasing significantly is lung cancer. Were it not for lung cancer, the combined incidence of all cancers among white males would be *decreasing*.

Of particular interest is the considerable decline in stomach cancer during the last half-century, as well as a less dramatic decrease in cancers of the colon and rectum. If processed foods were guilty of causing or contributing to the development of cancer, it is those very sites that one would expect to be most affected.

One cannot help wondering if food processing might not have had precisely the opposite effect: Perhaps it is something put *into* our food that tends to inhibit cancer development.

A few years ago a prominent television "news" show created a national stir by blatantly misinforming the public that the United States was "number one" in cancer.* Then as now the

* CBS Reports Special, "The American Way of Cancer," hosted by Dan Rather, October 15, 1975.

MALE CANCER DEATH RATES* BY SITE
UNITED STATES, 1930-1978

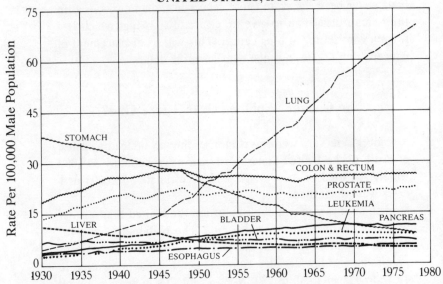

FEMALE CANCER DEATH RATES* BY SITE
UNITED STATES, 1930-1978

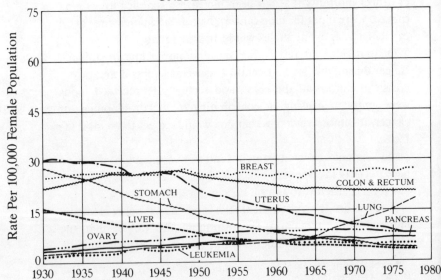

*Rates for male and female populations standardized for age
on the 1970 U.S. population

Sources of Data: National Vital Statistics Division and
Bureau of the Census, United States

Epidemiology & Statistics Dept. American Cancer Society, 6-81

actual statistics, easily available, tell us that the United States ranks *21st* in a list of 44 developed countries worldwide.* The dubious distinction of "number one" belongs to Scotland, with an annual male death rate of 205 per 100,000 persons compared to the United States male death rate of 157 per 100,000. Other countries with higher cancer death rates than the United States include such geographically varied ones as France, Italy, Uruguay, Australia, Denmark, Czechoslovakia, as well as the British crown colony of Hong Kong.

How a supposedly competent agency could so thoroughly misconstrue the data given their reporter is astonishing indeed. Nevertheless, passing numbers around is of little more than academic interest if you or someone dear to you has been touched by cancer. The basic concern is not how much cancer we *don't* have, but how much we do have and what is being done about it.

WHY DO WE KNOW SO LITTLE?

It is grossly unfair to the field of medical research to assume we know very little about cancer. Actually, we know a great deal. The problem, of course, is how much more there is that we do not know. And in most cases, the area is too complex to be able to apply what is learned about skin cancer, for instance, to such vastly different forms of the disease as breast cancer or leukemia.

The research has been extensive and continues to be so, but, as with heart disease, scientists are constantly having to struggle with the frustrations of conflicting evidence. In dealing with the role of diet in disease, we know even less about the diet-cancer link than we do about diet and heart disease. And that means that at this moment we know very little indeed.

We do know that some kind of association exists—at least for some forms of the disease. Populations with different dietary patterns generally exhibit differing cancer patterns. Interestingly, as persons emigrate from one country to another and adapt their eating habits to those of the new country, they eventually also

* World Health Statistics Annual, 1972–1973. The figures are based on the number of deaths per 100,000 population.

assume the health and disease patterns, cancer included, of the adopted country. For instance, Japanese living in Japan have higher rates of stomach cancer and lower rates of breast cancer than are found in the United States. But Japanese who have migrated to this country gradually develop cancer-incidence patterns increasingly similar to those of the United States; that is, the incidence of stomach cancer declines while that of breast cancer climbs.

Generally speaking, the drawbacks of relying on human subjects in cancer studies are manifold, and most of them are obvious. (There is a striking shortage of volunteers, for one thing.) Consequently, scientists traditionally employ test animals for their investigations, a situation not without limitations. To begin with, there are considerable metabolic and physiological differences between humans and other animals, and we can never be entirely sure that man will be affected by any given substance in the same way as another species.

Next is the question of dosage. The enormous amounts of a suspected carcinogen (cancer-causing substance) fed or injected into laboratory animals have created a wealth of source material for humorists. But it is not quite as silly as it sounds. The relatively short lifespan of the usual species of test animals necessitates doses high enough to initiate observable reactions—if there are going to be any—before the creatures succumb to old age. Levels are generally far beyond what would normally be consumed in the human diet.

Dosage level, biological differences, and other potential variables present monumental problems when one is trying to extrapolate results in such a way that they become meaningful to the life-styles of humans. Moreover, interpretations are never specific. At the same time one group of experts is concluding that a particular set of data is significant, an equally knowledgeable group is sure to insist that it is not.

To further complicate the investigations, studies of the same suspected carcinogen do not always agree with one another. One study may show a positive correlation, others may show none at all, and still others may even show an inverse relationship. For instance, in the researching of cereals and other grain products, as many studies indicate that these foods may *prevent* cancer as have shown that they may *cause* cancer (and additional studies have revealed no association, either negative or positive). Similarly, contradictory results have been obtained with such foods as fish, and various vegetables and fruits. There is simply no way to draw accurate conclusions from such conflicting evidence— even when all the research is conducted in accordance with the principles of the scientific method and uses a significantly large sampling.

While all of this may be perplexing to the consumer, it is only fair to assume it is even more so to the scientists who have been so desperately searching for answers.

THE ''AUTHORITIES'' SPEAK

In spite of the need for a cautious approach to the interpretation of animal test results, there are those who snatch a few pieces of the puzzle and present them to the public as the total picture. As any jigsaw fan knows, nothing could be more deceptive.

In March of 1979, Dr. Guy R. Newell, deputy director of the National Cancer Institute (NCI), stated that although there was no proof, "information" suggested that increased dietary fiber might help reduce the risk of colon cancer, and therefore we should all eat more fresh fruits and vegetables.*

By October 1979, Dr. Arthur Upton, then director of the NCI, publicly expanded the fiber theory and advised all Americans that to reduce the risk of developing cancer, they should not only eat more fiber, but they should also eat less fat, drink less alcohol, and avoid being overweight. He went on to note that his recommendations were based on "incomplete evidence," but that

---

* The theory had its roots, of course, in Burkitt's African studies discussed in chapter 3: the contention that increased "bulk" could perhaps prevent colon cancer, which later became the basis for the "Save-Your-Life" and other bran diets.

175

we should abide by what he termed "prudent interim principles."

Critics insist it is highly unlikely that Dr. Upton would have offered his recommendations without pressure from Senator George McGovern. Up to that time, all of the National Institutes of Health (NIH), of which NCI is only one branch, had maintained that the available scientific evidence was simply not yet convincing enough to warrant overall dietary changes as a means of prevention for *any* major disease. No significant breakthrough, which might have influenced his position, had occurred at the time of Upton's statement. McGovern, however, had been advocating the need for dietary change ever since publication of his ill-advised *Dietary Goals for the United States* in 1977. The goals set the National Institutes of Health in a bad light, a situation that they have since attempted to remedy without changing their basic stand on the issues.

In spite of extensive criticism by renowned experts, the power-wielding McGovern stubbornly refused to change his position on what he personally viewed as changes necessary to the American diet. But the shaky claims of his dietary goals needed some sort of corroboration, and evidently the NIH was his focal point for attack. For starters, McGovern voiced extreme criticism of the methods NIH used for allocating research grants, citing insufficient "peer review" and threatening to launch a full-scale investigation by the General Accounting Office.* While NIH officials turned up their collective noses at McGovern's allegations, there was—as there always is—the nuisance of having to contend with work disrupted during such investigations.

Daniel S. Greenberg in his "Washington Report" column commented at length upon the pressure forced on Upton, noting: "It is doubtful that this statement would have been issued without McGovern's insistence. Whether the public will be better off for it is something that won't be known for a long time, if ever." However indirectly, the knuckling-under of the National Cancer Institute represents yet another consequence of the political

* This is a strange cry, indeed, considering that McGovern himself was accused of this same omission upon publication of *Dietary Goals.*

power struggle. McGovern's maneuvers to "prove" himself right can at this time have only one effect: a misinformed public.

In contrast to Dr. Upton's NCI declaration, the Surgeon General's report, *Healthy People,* which appeared at about the same time, was far more conservative in its statements: "The precise relationship between dietary differences and various cancers is still not known." The report further noted that "the association between diet and cancer is more tenuous than between diet and heart disease."

The current status of information on the diet-cancer link is even more succinctly summarized by the statements of two prominent medical scientists. Dr. Peter Greenwald, director of the Division of Epidemiology at the New York State Department of Health, in addressing the American Health Foundation, remarked:

The hypotheses relating diet to cancer are complex. . . . A convergence of evidence from different disciplines suggests strongly that diet is related to several common cancers, but we need further research before we have any consensus on the mechanisms or the proportion of cancers for which diet plays a role.

And the late Dr. Michael Halberstam, former editor of *Modern Medicine,* indicated that while there are some clues implicating dietary patterns in the development of some forms of cancer, the picture is far from clear:

The epidemiology of colon cancer seems associated with fat in the diet, but the association is so tenuous, so interwoven with a dozen other individual and social factors . . . no reputable scientist considers it other than a hypothesis.

We concur with the judgment of both of these well-respected individuals.

The Dietary Suspects

The cause of the increase in lung cancer is well understood: cigarette smoking. The decline in stomach cancer is less clear. Some scientists feel it results from a wider use of refrigeration and the addition of preservatives—particularly antioxidants—in our food supply. On the other hand, national surveys show that a large number of Americans believe that "chemicals" added to our foods present a serious cancer hazard. Their fears are understandable in light of all the recent scare headlines concerning artificial sweeteners, preservatives, and coloring agents. But as we noted in the last chapter, popular wisdom is not supported by scientific facts.

Although scientists have been unable to demonstrate any *direct* cause/effect relationship between diet and cancer, they do know that various associations exist. Perhaps the balance and type of nutrients in the diet may in some way influence cancer development by altering the environment of tissue cells that are already susceptible to malignant change. Similarly, nutrient intake might also affect certain biological processes, which could in turn trigger tumor formation.

In other words, present indications are that in some persons nutrition may influence an existing susceptibility, either of a hereditary nature or resulting from other factors.

FATS AND CHOLESTEROL

Cancer of the breast is the leading cancer killer of American women. Cancer of the colon is the second leading cause of cancer death for both males and females. Prostate cancer is the third most common form of cancer death in men, and, if it were not for cigarette smoking, it would be vying with colon cancer for the number-one position among men.

Something has to explain these very significant differences between our rates of cancer and those, for instance, of Japanese in

178

Japan. Arguments that some nationalities are genetically "prone" to certain cancers are not very convincing, because people moving from a low-risk country to a high-risk country do not retain low risks. As an example, second-generation Japanese women in the United States have a breast-cancer pattern much the same as the national average, even though in their native land this disease is relatively uncommon. Other factors such as occupation and childbearing methods can be similarly ruled out.

Japanese in Japan, however, do eat differently from Americans. The former build their diets around fish, rice, and vegetables, and their intake of fat averages only about 12 percent of total calories. Americans tend to eat more meats, eggs, and dairy products, with some 40 percent of dietary calories accounted for by fat. Like other migrants, the longer they continue to live in our country, the more likely the Japanese are to follow the eating patterns of their new homeland.

As shown in the chart below, other less affluent countries and those following "non-Western" diets also have low rates of colon, breast, and prostate cancer. Countries with eating patterns similar to ours (such as Australia, Canada, and Denmark) have high rates of these diseases. In addition, blacks who live in rural parts of the United States have a lower incidence of cancer of the colon than do blacks living in cities, presumably because in many areas, rural dwellers are less affluent and eat different foods.

But current evidence of the link between cancer and diet is not nearly as strong as are other links in the development of human malignancy. Nevertheless, if the relationship is at all valid it should hold up under cross-examination. It would follow, then, that groups of individuals living in the United States but following a low-fat dietary pattern should have lower rates of cancer of the breast, prostate, and colon. Seventh Day Adventists do use fatty foods relatively less frequently and do have only slightly more than half the national cancer rate. On the other hand, Mormons suffer only 60 to 75 percent as much cancer as the national average and consume about the same amount of fat as do other Americans.

179

Figure 3
Selected Cancer Death Rates Around the World 1976–77*

	Breast	Prostate Gland	Colon and Rectum Male	Colon and Rectum Female	Stomach Male	Stomach Female
Group #1						
United States	27.3	22.3	26.2	20.2	9.2	4.4
Australia	24.8	21.9	33.4	22.5	15.7	8.4
Canada	28.4	21.0	28.6	23.0	15.8	7.2
Denmark	33.8	21.1	28.6	25.9	19.0	9.7
Group #2						
Costa Rica	11.4	15.3	8.2	8.4	61.1	38.8
Bulgaria	14.6	8.9	13.5	9.4	36.6	20.3
Japan	5.7	3.6	15.0	11.1	70.2	34.9

* Annual age-adjusted death rate per 100,000 population.
Source: American Cancer Society: Cancer Facts and Figures—1982.

And animal studies do not always support the hypothesis that fat may be involved in cancer causation. Specifically, research has raised the question of whether it is the amount of specific *kinds* of fats that is the influencing factor. While conclusions are inconsistent and sometimes ambiguous, there is a very definite trend linking polyunsaturated fatty acids with tumor formation in animals.

The possibility exists that nutrition may influence the development of cancers of the breast, ovary, uterus, and prostate by changing hormonal status and balance. Circumstantial evidence implicating nutrition has led to a number of hypotheses that are still being tested. For example, some scientists propose that a dietary influence on hormones reduces the age at which menarche takes place, which hormonal change could increase one's vulnerability to breast cancer. Native-born Americans do mature earlier than in previous generations. Maximum growth, which is closely associated with onset of maturity, is one of the major health goals in the United States. Along with this emphasis on achieving maximum height, the maturation age has been lowered. If it is indeed true that early maturation due to hormone modification through nutrition is linked with cancer, then health goals may have to be modified. But none of this is settled. Much more study is required.

LACK OF FIBER

Dr. Denis Burkitt, a surgeon who spent many of his years of practice in Africa, is convinced that the lack of dietary fiber (also known as "roughage" or "bulk") is a major cause of several common diseases in developed countries, among them cancer of the colon. He and others have emphasized that a high-fiber diet, as opposed to one which consists mainly of highly processed foods, offers protection from colon cancer by increasing stool volume and promoting a more rapid "transit time" for the feces. He suggests that when the bowel is exposed to stools for a longer period of time, the organ is irritated and possibly exposed to potentially cancer-causing agents for a prolonged period.

Burkitt's high-fiber diet has already been mentioned in chapter 3 on weight control. And while many Americans have been wishfully stuffing themselves with bran as a means of quick weight loss, just as many are doing exactly the same in the hope of preventing cancer. At this point, however, the idea remains just one of many hypotheses and contains some serious gaps. For example, there is no evidence of increased risk of colon cancer in individuals who chronically suffer from constipation, an observation that casts doubt on the "transit time" theory. Furthermore, experiments with diet modification in animals do not support the notion that high-fiber diets offer protection from cancer.

Additionally, there is no strong evidence correlating the fiber content of foods with the incidence of colon cancer in countries around the world.

OBESITY

Obesity is considered to be a risk factor for both breast and uterine cancer. According to Dr. John W. Berg from the Cancer Epidemiology Research Center at the University of Iowa: "Endometrial [uterine] cancer is the one cancer in this country consistently associated with obesity." Other researchers point out that this association has not always been confirmed, but it must nevertheless be noted that uterine cancer is one of the health risks of too much weight.

ALCOHOL

Alcohol alone has never been shown to cause cancer in either animals or humans. There is reason to believe, however, that heavy drinkers—particularly those who also smoke cigarettes—are at greater risk of developing cancer of the esophagus, larynx, oral cavity, and liver.

Dr. Kenneth Rothman from the Harvard School of Public Health calculates that if you smoke two packs of cigarettes a day, you increase the risk of oral cancer by 143 percent compared with a nonsmoker. If you also have just two drinks a day, your risk skyrockets to almost *1,500 percent.* That's a good case against excessive drinking, particularly if you're also a smoker (and we wholeheartedly recommend that you keep away from cigarettes).

VITAMINS AND MINERALS

Research has been under way to test the effects of various nutrients in relation to cancer. There are indications that vitamins C and E might possibly have a blocking action against certain cancer-causing agents, but a number of studies have failed to support the theory.

Nutrient testing can become complex in the extreme. As an example, bracken fern, a popular salad food in such countries as Japan, contains a naturally occurring carcinogen. It also contains an enzyme that destroys thiamine, a B vitamin. Researchers logically assumed that a thiamine supplement would counteract the cancer-causing effect, but, completely opposite to their expectations, supplements of thiamine actually *increased* the development of tumors.

Recent evidence from the National Cancer Institute indicates that certain vitamin deficiencies tend to promote tumor development, while other deficiencies suppress it. Further, excessive intake of vitamins can influence tumor development in *either* direction. Similarly, most minerals appear to have an optimum range for consumption. Either too little or too much may increase tumor formation or the susceptibility to some other cancer-causing agent.

VEGETABLES AND FRUITS

Investigations attempting to establish a relationship between cancer and the vegetable/fruit family have led only to opposing results. However, the most recent research reveals the possible inhibitory effects of certain chemicals known as indoles. These indoles occur naturally in cabbage, broccoli, cauliflower, brussels sprouts, turnips, and other members of the cabbage family. While there are no claims that indoles actually prevent cancer, the theory is that they may have the ability to inhibit cancer-cell growth in both the breast and colon.

Still other plant chemicals that may produce similar blocking effects are coumarins, constituents of a wide variety of both vegetables and fruits. At the time of this writing, however, the anti-cancer properties of neither indoles nor coumarins have been established. Continuing research should eventually lead to firmer results.

DIETS OF OTHER COUNTRIES

The incidence of stomach cancer for both men and women in the United States has declined by more than 50 percent during the last quarter-century. Our current death rate from this disease is one-third that of thirty years ago. In attempting to uncover the reasons why our country has been comparatively fortunate in this respect, it is useful to take a look at dietary differences in such countries as Japan, which has a male rate of stomach cancer of 62 per 100,000 individuals as compared to 8 in the United States.

One possibility is the excessively high salt consumption among the Japanese. A great many everyday dishes are prepared with soy sauce, soybean paste, and salted pickles and fish. These food items may contain as much as 20 percent salt—far more than anyone needs.

A favorite Japanese technique for preparing fish (for instance, in teriyaki) involves salting and drying it, and then broiling it until it is burned black. Rice is sometimes prepared in much the same way. Cold rice is often formed into balls and baked until the surface is burned slightly black and becomes as hard as glass. Only recently have carcinogenic substances been isolated from the charred portions of these and other commonly eaten foods.

In other countries with high rates of stomach cancer—Costa Rica and Bulgaria, for instance—food-preparation methods may also play a role, particularly the use of smoking as a preservative. Primitive means of food storage that allow it to become contaminated may very well add to the problem.

Interestingly enough, while the United States as a whole has a very low rate of stomach cancer, there are certain "hot spots" with unusually high rates of this disease. There is an impressive cluster of stomach cancer in certain rural counties of the north-central region of the nation (Minnesota, the Dakotas, Michigan, and Wisconsin). Concentrated in these areas are people of Russian, Austrian, Scandinavian, and German descent. The susceptibility of these ethnic groups to stomach cancer might be compatible with the fact that there is also a high incidence of the disease in their native lands. Moreover, this type of clustering provides another clue. While the dietary patterns of these areas are still under study, a common theme has already emerged: a large proportion of highly spiced, smoked food. However, if dietary patterns or other behaviors changed among these people, we might also see a decrease in cancer. This seems to be the case with Japanese who have come to the United States; the second generation has a lower incidence of stomach cancer.

Fortunately, smoked, heavily salted, highly spiced foods do not regularly comprise a large portion of the average American diet. There is no reason to suspect that charcoal-broiled hamburgers or steaks will introduce substantial amounts of carcinogens into our systems. Actually, highly salted, smoked, and burnt foods have not been confirmed as direct causes of stomach cancer, in any case.

"Health-Food" Treatments—Organic and Otherwise

For a long time now the health-food industry has been busily cashing in on the almost universal fear of cancer. The array of cures and preventatives outnumber even the many forms of cancer; yet each is usually dubbed a cure-all. In some cases we must assume the intentions are honorable, but the same fallacy occurs over and over: A shred of inconclusive information is used to build a theory, but there is no solid foundation to support it.

We hear about the marvels of beet juices, onions, calves' liver, raw milk, bran, and every conceivable "wonder food" and vitamin/mineral preparation. If someone hasn't already suggested you eat more cabbage ("organic," of course), you're bound to hear it sooner or later.

VITAMINS

Dr. Linus Pauling, not content merely to cure the common cold with vitamin C, has also suggested that his favorite supervitamin will also cure cancer. This hypothesis is apparently based on certain animal studies that indicate vitamin C can inhibit the formation of nitrosamines in the stomach and large intestine. But again, other studies show no anticancer effects attributed to vitamin C.

Dr. Michael Sporn of the National Cancer Institute recently discussed the possible preventive effects of a vitamin A derivative known as 13-cis retinoic acid. Specifically, the chemical is being tested among persons who are at very high risk of developing bladder cancer, but there are indications that it may also be able to inhibit cancer of the lung, breast, esophagus, pancreas, and colon. However, just because "vitamin A" was mentioned in this connection is no reason to start taking vitamin A tablets. In fact, if vitamin A is taken in excess, it will accumulate and can be toxic. Also, 13-cis retinoic acid is *not* vitamin A but a similar chemical compound, and the product is only at the testing stage.

ARTIFICIAL ADDITIVES

Of course, a favorite argument by the health foodist is that most of America's cancer is caused by food additives, and that we can all expect to live longer, healthier lives if we confine ourselves to "natural" eating. Results of some of the lopsided studies conducted with additives during the past few years might at first glance appear to support the idea. But other countries, such as Poland and Czechoslovakia, which seldom use American means of food preservation have overall cancer rates similar to or higher than those of the United States. There just is no convincing evidence that chemicals added to food substantially increase the risk of any form of human cancer. Indeed, the facts are directly contrary. Specifically, referring to figures 1 and 2 at the beginning of this chapter, the decline in the incidence of gastrointestinal cancers during the past fifty to sixty years suggests that something added to our food supply is helping to *prevent* the development of these forms of cancer, most likely the various antioxidants such as BHA and BHT.

Again, while most research in this area is still sketchy and somewhat contradictory, new studies conducted with both animals and people indicate that BHA and BHT (butylated hydroxyanisole and butylated hydroxytoluene), which are used in minute amounts as food additives, may possess anticancer properties. Both compounds are antioxidants that are frequently used as preservatives in such products as cereal and baked goods. BHT in very high doses is too toxic to be considered a possible therapeutic agent against cancer, but BHA may have important future uses. According to Dr. Lee Wattenberg of the University of Minnesota, the substance has been demonstrated to effectively block nitrosamine formation, as well as the action of other carcinogens, including those believed to be involved in cancers related to cigarette smoking.

The obvious question that arises is why these cancer-inhibiting substances are not immediately prescribed for general use. The reason is simply that not enough is known about them yet. A great deal more research is necessary before levels can be established that are high enough to be effective but low enough to be free of side effects. Whether any of the compounds mentioned here will ever prove to be of value for most people is still to be determined.

In spite of the promising anticancer future of certain food additives and naturally occurring food chemicals, we continue to recommend caution—and common sense! Investigative results are still premature. It is hoped that some of these substances will eventually serve to reduce cancer rates. But we remind you once again of the need for moderation. As yet there is no way of knowing the point at which the "cure" might be worse than the disease.

Cancer Quackery

No discussion of cancer and diet would be complete without mention of the blatant types of quackery that have been employed by the unscrupulous. Among health foodists, we frequently encounter self-"cures" that have been used to treat self-diagnosed diseases. Naturally, any doctor or would-be doctor is aware of the ease with which one can eliminate a condition that does not exist in the first place: Any treatment at all would constitute an effective "cure."

Cancer, because so little is known about it in comparison to other major diseases, is a field ripe for every sort of quackery. A sure way to begin sifting out frauds is when you notice: a) They are recommended only by their own patients, whom they have diagnosed, treated, and "cured"; or b) they lament the fact that their methods are not accepted in legitimate medical circles (with good reason!); or c) they claim a "secret" cure (reminiscent of that favorite office slogan that explains: "My work is so secret I don't even know what I'm doing").

187

LAETRILE

During the past few years the most notable phony cancer cure to hit the public bears the commercial name of Laetrile. Chemically, the substance is known as amygdalin, sometimes also referred to as "aprikern" (because it is derived from the pits of stone-bearing fruits, principally apricots) or "vitamin B_{17}." This last term is particularly ludicrous in that the American Institute of Nutrition's Committee on Nomenclature has found no scientific evidence for the existence of any such vitamin as B_{17}—a fact that ought to create immediate suspicion. Cancer is sometimes accused of being a deficiency disease, but most assuredly it is not caused by a deficiency of a nonexistent vitamin.

The hypothesis behind Laetrile is based on the presumed release of cyanide resulting from the enzymatic action of cancer cells on the amygdalin. Not only is the process totally ineffective against cancer-cell destruction, but if Laetrile is administered by mouth it can result in cyanide poisoning.

Repeated studies have been conducted at reputable medical research institutes in an attempt to determine the validity of Laetrile's rave notices. Continually, the substance has proved worthless, and the testimonials themselves have been shown to be based on incomplete case histories. Yet pro-Laetrile arguments still abound. As one example of several delusive books on the market, *Laetrile Case Histories,* by John A. Richardson, M.D., and Patricia Griffin, R.N., describes "ninety actual case histories that reveal for the first time how Laetrile has been used in the treatment of cancer at the Richardson Cancer Clinic, Berkeley, California."

For several years Laetrile has been easily obtained in Mexico, even though it was illegal in the United States until 1978. At that time, the drug was federally approved for cancer patients who had been medically certified as "terminally ill." By fall of that year, seventeen states had legalized Laetrile, but it was still prohibited from interstate commerce, thus rendering it basically inaccessible, for all practical purposes. The supreme hoax is that the drug costs only about two cents per pill to produce but sells for anywhere from $1.25 a pill and up. The latest available figures reveal that an estimated 70,000 Americans are now using this totally useless drug.

A few media personnel have unwittingly aided the spread of some of the wonder stories about Laetrile. Sensationalism will always find an audience, and windmill chasers would apparently as soon turn to Laetrile as any other miracle worker. That many have become convinced they need daily supplements of Laetrile to avoid cancer is simply a flagrant waste of money. But the others, the cancer patients who have been persuaded to forego legitimate medical treatment, and perhaps expensive surgery, in favor of a worthless noncure—they are the real victims. Few who have been stricken by cancer can afford time for such life-draining mistakes.

As we go to press, the *New England Journal of Medicine* published the results of a large clinical trial of Laetrile in the treatment of human cancer and concluded, "Laetrile is a toxic drug that is not effective as a cancer treatment." In an accompanying editorial, Dr. Arnold Relman wrote, "Laetrile, I believe, has now had its day in court. The evidence, beyond reasonable doubt, is that it doesn't benefit patients with advanced cancer, and there is no reason to believe it would be any more effective in the earlier stages of the disease. Some, undoubtedly, will remain unconvinced, but no sensible person will want to advocate its further use, and no state legislature should sanction it any longer. The time has come to close the books on Laetrile and get on with our efforts to understand the riddle of cancer and improve its prevention and treatment."

OTHER NONCURES

Unfortunately, Laetrile is only one in a long parade of quack treatments for cancer. The list is far too extensive to mention here more than one or two. One longtime favorite, Krebiozen, was supposedly obtained from the blood of horses that had received special injections. In reality, the concoction consisted primarily of mineral oil. Other treatments over the years have employed the use of laxatives, salves, and various drugs, with or without the addition of special foods.

One of the most notorious pseudo-cures is a substance known as "glyoxylide," introduced several decades ago by Dr. William F. Koch of the Detroit Medical College, now defunct. Authorities very soon became aware that glyoxylide injections were worthless, but they were unable to prosecute Koch for twenty years. The reason? Dr. Koch's glyoxylide was merely water, and therefore harmless. (Today's laws are, of course, much more stringent.)

Incredible as it may seem, this nontreatment still has its proponents, who claim the only reason glyoxylide didn't work for others was because it wasn't used in conjunction with the prescribed diet. Ronald Deutsch, in his book *The New Nuts Among the Berries* (1977), notes that some cancer quacks still administer glyoxylide injections and that these injections were shown to cost anywhere from $25 to $300 each—a juicy profit for plain water. (And it doesn't even have any ocean water in it.)

The Dilemma

We in the scientific community are keenly aware of the indications that nutrition is involved in some way with some forms of cancer. The frustration is that we don't yet know precisely how.

Cancer is a frightening proposition. We all want answers *now*—and they are just not available yet. Authors, government officials, media people, and the health-food industry know only too well that people in the grip of fear are willing to listen to almost anything. We can only caution you once again not to get carried away by unsubstantiated theories or ideas that are based only on preliminary, incomplete data without regard for possible adverse effects. Cancer requires sound diagnosis, and the best we have in treatment—medical surgical, and chemical—not quack recommendations.

Until the cancer-diet association becomes much clearer than it is today, our dietary advice is the same as for heart disease:

1) Don't make major dietary changes unless they are recommended by a well-qualified physician after a medical diagnosis.
2) Eat a well-balanced diet, but only in amounts such that you reach and then maintain your Desirable Weight.

As this book went to press, a committee of the National Academy of Sciences issued a report, *Diet, Nutrition and Cancer,* which reviewed the complex scientific literature in this field, and made some specific dietary recommendations, implying that they would be helpful in decreasing one's chances of developing cancer.

The NAS report's "interim dietary guidelines" advised Americans

- To reduce dietary fat intake from the current level of about 40 percent of total calories to 30 percent of total calories.
- To include fruits, vegetables, and whole grain cereal products in the daily diet. (This, of course, is good general nutrition advice.) Citrus fruits, carotene-rich vegetables, and cruciferous (cabbage family) vegetables were particularly recommended.
- To minimize consumption of salt-cured, salt-pickled, and smoked foods.
- To consume alcoholic beverages in moderation, if one chooses to consume them at all. (Good general health advice.)

Our views on *Diet, Nutrition and Cancer* were well-stated by our colleague at the American Council on Science and Health, Dr. Alfred E. Harper, professor of biochemistry and nutrition at the University of Wisconsin, and former chairman of the Food and Nutrition Board of the National Academy of Sciences.

In an interview with the *New York Times,* Dr. Harper said,

"We don't know enough about diet and cancer to make recommendations that will either create hopes that are unlikely to be fulfilled or create apprehension because of the inability to achieve the recommendations."

It is also of interest to note that the very last sentence of the thick NAS report is as follows: "However, the Committee concluded that the data are not sufficient to quantitate the contribution of diet to overall cancer risk or to determine the percent reduction in risk that might be achieved by dietary modification." So why all the fuss?

CHAPTER 7

Sugar: The Killer on the Breakfast Table?

Accusations Against Sugar

Propaganda of recent years has pronounced sugar one of the world's most fearsome ingredients—right up there with the Black Plague. "Sugar and spice and everything nice," once a complimentary tag for very young ladies, is greeted today with paternal frowns. Sweetness is anathema. A dash of fructose may be acceptable, but that's the absolute outer limit.

The accusations are rampant. We are told that sugar causes everything from constipation to learning disabilities. No one, from infant to centenarian, is immune from its deadly attack. The substance is allegedly responsible for a Pandora's box full of chronic diseases and other maladies.

The U.S. government stands ready to "help." Soon after the McGovern Committee dubbed sugar an unnecessary evil in "Dietary Goals," the Federal Trade Commission drew up a set of recommendations to ban the advertising of sugary products during children's television shows. (Fortunately, the FTC recently dropped this recommendation.) And the U.S. Department of Agriculture proposed that sales of snack foods and soft drinks in schools be forbidden. (This, too, has been dropped, and wisely.) A few food processors have joined the forces. "No sugar added!" scream the TV commercials. "Only Mother Nature's own sweetener!" proclaim the magazine ads. "Sugar-free," boast the food labels. People have begun to brag that they no longer use the substance, as though that were a virtue. (Such abstention calls to mind all the people who "never" watch television. Except documentaries.)

All of this apprehension and misinformation is based on two false premises: The first is that Americans are consuming more sugar today than ever before. The second is the mistaken notion that modern sugar consumption contributes to poor health. Neither statement is even remotely true.

CONSUMPTION STATISTICS

Government statistics reveal very little change in American sugar consumption over the past half-century. According to the U.S. Department of Agriculture, the average person consumed 104.3 pounds per year of sugar during 1925, an amount that declined gradually, though not steadily, to 97.6 pounds in 1960. By 1970, annual consumption was up again to 101.9 pounds,* followed by another decline to 79.5 pounds in 1981.

Of course, you don't need a computer to tell you that these figures still average out to slightly less than two pounds of sugar per week per person, and at first thought that does seem like a lot. But those two pounds merit a fuller explanation. First, they include the sugar from all sugar-containing products we eat, in-

* The Food and Drug Administration Select Committee on GRAS (Generally Recognized as Safe) Substances put the 1970 consumption figure at 102.5 pounds. That calculates to approximately half a percent difference, which is not a significant deviation.

cluding such items as catsup and mayonnaise. Second, the figures are based on *disappearance* data, rather than on actual consumption.

Disappearance, in other words, refers to total shipments of sugar without taking into account any loss or spoilage, what may be disposed of in the kitchen sink or garbage can, or used in fermentation where the sugar is changed to carbon dioxide and escapes as a gas. Leading research authorities, including the USDA, the Select Committee on GRAS Substances, and the National Research Council, estimate that actual sugar *consumption* is between 20 and 25 percent *less* than the disappearance data indicates. In addition to an unknown amount of spillage and waste, considerable sugar disappears by way of the fermentation processes in bread baking, for example, or in making other food ingredients.

Further, when considered in proportion to total dietary intake, the two-pound figure is not inordinately high. A pound of sugar contains 1,748 calories. Calculated as a percentage of total energy (i.e., calorie) intake, the numbers come into clearer perspective: In 1974, sugar consumption—even based on disappearance data—represented only 14.1 percent of total calorie intake, a figure well within the range acceptable to most nutrition authorities. Even McGovern's "Dietary Goals" proposes that the American diet consist of 15 percent sugar.

Where "Dietary Goals" is in error, however, is in its contention that our current diet is comprised of 24 percent sugar, rather than an amount closer to 14 percent. Although the figure implies that it refers to common refined white sugar (sucrose), it in fact also includes other diverse forms of sugar that occur naturally in foods, like milk, fruit, syrups, and honey. The comparison is not only inaccurate; it is unfair and unrealistic.

KINDS AND FORMS OF SUGAR—WHAT IT IS

Of course, the health faddists are quick to complain that it is only refined white sugar that is dangerous; "natural" sweeteners are just fine, even good for us. Before deciding on the truth of such claims, let's first take a closer look at just what we—and they—are talking about.

Chemically, there are a great many compounds that are called sugars, but only a few of these are found in the foods we eat. Most common of these are *sucrose,* or common table sugar, which is derived from either cane or beet sugar; *glucose,* the sugar found in our blood; *fructose,* sometimes called "fruit sugar"; and *lactose,* a sugar found in milk. Both glucose and fructose are extremely common in the plant world; vegetables and fruits with a sweet taste generally contain varying amounts of sucrose as well. (In the case of sugarcane, for instance, the plants contain more sucrose than any other sugar.) In order to be used by the body, all sugars must ultimately be converted to glucose, and the human body cares little where its supplies originate. Additionally, all other carbohydrates—such as starch—must first be converted to glucose before they can be of any use to the body.

Sugars readily connect and disconnect themselves into chains of molecules that vary in length. Sucrose is easily separated into glucose and fructose. Conversely, glucose and fructose combine to form sucrose. Honey is composed of all three of these sugars. Thus, when we hear of honey as a nutritionally superior sweetener, as man has been hearing through the ages, the statement is simply untrue. Whether the sucrose is separated into glucose and fructose before we swallow it or afterwards is not a matter of importance to good health. Honey does contain minute amounts of nutrients other than sugars, but these minute amounts are nutritionally insignificant. Honey also contains nonnutrient compounds (nasty old chemicals) that give it its distinctive, enjoyable flavor.

Similarly, a great deal is heard these days about the wonderful properties of fructose. The health-food stores are particularly fond of pushing it on their customers. In reality, fructose is somewhat sweeter than ordinary sugar, so it is true that less is required to achieve the same level of sweetness. But extracting natural fructose from fruits is very expensive. Recently, most commercial fructose has been processed enzymatically from corn starch at greatly reduced costs. Fructose must still be converted to glucose by the digestive system before it enters the blood. The before-or-after question here becomes not only moot but downright silly. Nevertheless, healthfoodland devotees continue to pay higher prices for a sugar that in essence has been partially predigested, calling it more "natural" while disallowing the body to perform a perfectly normal function.

Theoretically, fructose may have one advantage for diabetics, since it requires less insulin than sucrose during metabolism, but this has little practical significance. We caution against the indiscriminate use of fructose by diabetics without a physician's approval. One problem is that the liver can also use fructose to make triglycerides (the technical term for fats), and some evidence suggests that fructose is more rapidly converted to fat than glucose.

NATURAL BROWN VS. NATURAL WHITE

Another antisugar cry is the claim that the refining process robs white sugar of its nutrients, leaving behind only "empty calories." Actually, empty calories do not exist; only food calories, food energy—4 calories per gram! It is true that refined sugar contains no vitamins, minerals, or protein, but that is not its purpose in the diet. Sugar in any form adds flavor. Since it is rarely eaten alone, it renders more palatable many foods that are rich in the nutrients sugar lacks. For example, ice cream is a mixture of milk, fat, and sugars. Or cake, a mixture of wheat, milk, eggs, fat, and sugar. Sweeteners are intended to complement, not replace, other items in the diet.

Sugar is not sold in its completely raw state, although health-food stores often sell turbinado sugar as "raw" sugar. Actually, turbinado has already been partially refined. Some of its original nutrients have been retained, but the amounts are too small to be important in one's total diet. The substance has a molasses flavor and is considerably less sweet than ordinary table sugar. It is not a very effective substitute for regular sugar, but nevertheless it is edible, if that is what you want to use as a sweetener and you are willing to pay the price for it.

Molasses is another extraction from sugar that is even less sweet than turbinado, although it contains slightly more vitamins and minerals. But if it's nutrients you're looking for rather than sweetness, you might as well go all the way with blackstrap molasses. Blackstrap has been described in one health-food publication as "the bottom of the barrel," and it is a fairly rich source of iron. But no one has to revert to eating this very unpalatable product. Much better-tasting foods are even better sources of iron; for example, meat. (The same publication cautions us to pay no attention to tales of blackstrap also containing "straw, dirt, and other extraneous material.")

Regular brown sugar, being less refined, is closer to white sugar in sweetening ability. Its distinctive flavor makes it desirable in many recipes, and some people prefer it for adding to breakfast cereals and other foods. Its reputation as being nutritionally superior to white sugar is, however, close to fiction. The traces of iron and B vitamins it possesses are nutritionally negligible.

SUGAR IS A FOOD

Sugars are digestible carbohydrates; therefore, they are food. In any reasonably well-balanced diet that includes a moderate amount of sugar, the average person receives all the nutrients needed and some to spare. Sugar is a tasty source of energy. It improves the flavor of a great many high-nutrient foods that would be far less tasty and certainly less interesting if left unsweetened. Further, sugar is a useful preservative, both commercially and in the home. Finally, Webster's Dictionary defines sugar as being "nutritionally important as a source of dietary carbohydrate and as a sweetener and preservative of other foods."

Whether in a refined form or in the original unrefined product, a molecule of sucrose is a molecule of sucrose. Whether the end product does or does not contain a whisper of riboflavin, for instance, has nothing whatever to do with the sucrose itself. More-over, the refining process does not *add* any undesirable sub-stances.

We would not presume to suggest what kind of sweetener you should be using. If you prefer the taste and texture of such prod-ucts as brown sugar or honey, by all means enjoy them. But what you must realize is that nutritionally you are achieving nothing by substituting these products for refined white sugar in your diet.

Misconceptions about Sugar

The popular misconceptions about sugar extend far beyond a vague, "It's-not-good-for-you." A number of specific charges have been circulated, most of which are groundless and contrary to scientific fact. Let's take a look at them.

O B E S I T Y

As discussed in chapter 3, excess calories, regardless of source, are fattening. No one kind of calorie is more fattening than any other. But one kind of energy *nutrient* (i.e., fat) does have a greater concentration of calories than the other two. All carbo-hydrates (including sugar) and all proteins contain about the same amount of calories per ounce. Fats contain more than twice the calories per ounce. Thus, an extra pat of butter or margarine on a slice of toast has more than twice the calories than an equal weight of sugar sprinkled on grapefruit or used in jelly or jam on bread.

Presumably, sugar was given this bad reputation because sweet desserts are among the first items to be eliminated from a reducing diet. This is done for two reasons: First, many sweet desserts are rich in fat as well as sugar, so that it is not the extra sugar alone that rings up that calorie score. A banana split, choc-olate mousse, or apple pie contains a high percentage of fat! Sec-ond, as any dieter knows, it takes a bit of juggling to maintain balanced menus with a limited number of calories. Rich desserts, no matter how "nutritious" they may be, contribute an excess number of calories in proportion to their vitamin-mineral-protein content—and it matters not at all whether those calories are sugar calories or fat calories. Perhaps we should refer more fairly to all those goodies as "fat-sweet desserts," rather than merely "sweet desserts." They certainly sound less appealing that way, which should be a plus for the dieter.

It makes no sense at all to attempt a sugar-free reducing diet if you replace the sugar with extra meat, sauces, gravies, french fries, and other fatty foods. A classic example is the obese person who makes a big thing about not putting sugar in his coffee after a four-course fatty meal. And wonders why he is gaining instead of losing.

DIABETES (MELLITUS)

Diabetes is the disease that results when the pancreas fails to produce enough insulin to maintain a normal level of blood sugar, i.e., glucose. The source of blood glucose is not only the diet; it also results from various metabolic processes in which fat and protein are converted to glucose. The normal concentration of glucose varies, depending upon when it is measured in relation to food intake. In diabetes, it is higher than normal, but high dietary intake or high blood sugar does not *cause* diabetes. Its cause is unknown.

For many years, diabetics were cautioned to curb their intake of all carbohydrates, including sugar, to keep their blood sugar from reaching dangerously high levels. By 1971, however, the Committee on Food and Nutrition for the American Diabetes Association advised a turnaround. Scientific data, they noted, revealed no apparent benefits from a disproportionate restriction of carbohydrates. Indeed, the data indicated exactly the opposite. First, the presence of sugar in the blood tends to *stimulate* additional insulin production. Second, a cutback in carbohydrates necessarily results in a greater proportion of protein and fat in the diet. And there is a well-documented direct relationship between diabetes, obesity, and arteriosclerosis; and an indirect association between obesity and heart disease.

Replacing carbohydrates with fatty foods is therefore not advisable for diabetics, especially those who are obese or tend to be so, since fat can easily be converted to glucose in the body. The American Diabetes Association emphasizes that, rather than eliminating any particular food group from the diet, the single most important objective is the prevention of obesity: "Adjustment of calories to attain or maintain optimal weight may be the most important part of dietary treatment and perhaps the only justified recommendation."

A word of caution: Diabetics must continue to avoid rapid ingestion of large amounts of sugar in order to prevent sudden surges in blood-sugar levels. But an *excess* of any food or nutrient is not recommended for anyone.

HYPOGLYCEMIA

The opposite of diabetes occurs when the pancreas produces too much insulin, resulting in blood-sugar levels that are abnormally low. This is called hypoglycemia (hypo = low; glycemia = sugar). Incidentally, neither sugar nor total carbohydrate consumption is a causative factor.

Misdiagnosed hypoglycemia is exceedingly popular these days. Some of the pseudo-scientific gurus would have us believe the condition has already reached epidemic proportions in the United States. The reason? A mammoth amount of self-diagnosis among the amateurs, and an almost equal amount of misdiagnosis and misinterpretation of test results among professionals. Add to this the ballyhoo in such current books as *Hypoglycemia: The Disease Your Doctor Won't Treat,* by Jeraldine Saunders and Harvey M. Ross, who erroneously complain, "Hypoglycemia is a condition often dismissed by the medical profession as a fad disease, over-diagnosed and very rare," and there is little wonder the public is somewhat confused.

In reality, true hypoglycemia (known as reactive hypoglycemia) is an extremely *rare* disease, with symptoms that display a remarkable parallel to those of anxiety neurosis. But how much easier it is to blame low blood sugar for one's inability or unwillingness to cope with the many problems of life.

Hypoglycemia is a handy scapegoat. It is tailor-made for hypochondriacs and an easy diagnosis for the patient who insists that a vague collection of symptoms be tagged with a name. You may feel we are suggesting that some physicians deliberately misdiagnose the condition in order to render prolonged expensive treatment, and you are absolutely correct. In all fairness, however, a mistaken diagnosis is frequently based on a misunderstanding of data and lack of sufficient knowledge about simple metabolism.

Few diseases can be diagnosed on the strength of symptoms alone, since so many symptoms are common to a great many physical ailments. To check for a malfunctioning of sugar metabolism, the medical profession uses what is known as the glucose tolerance test (GTT). The patient is usually instructed to eat or drink nothing after 7 P.M. the night before the test is to be conducted. The following morning, before breakfast, a fasting blood specimen is drawn as a control. Immediately after that, the patient must drink a specific amount of concentrated glucose solution. At hourly intervals thereafter, usually for five hours, additional blood samples are collected to determine how quickly and efficiently the patient's body is able to metabolize sugar; that is, bring the increased level down to near the fasting level of blood sugar.

The diabetic's blood may require the full five hours to return to normal sugar levels. In the true hypoglycemic, not only will the fasting specimen contain very little blood sugar, but after the glucose solution is swallowed, the blood sugar will return to normal rather quickly. In the latter part of the test, the sugar level will have fallen well below average, perhaps as low as 30 mg/100 ml or less.

What about the normal in-between person? The picture varies considerably, but almost always the blood sugar will be below average during the last one to three hours of the test. It is not surprising. Suppose the tolerance test is begun at 9 A.M. A five-hour test won't be completed until 2 P.M.—that's nineteen hours with nothing to eat except a little sugar water. We can safely assume the patient is *hungry*. And the body's blood-sugar level normally falls when we are hungry.

Indeed, it is believed by most authorities that this normal periodic fall in blood sugar is what triggers a reaction in an area of the hypothalamus section of the brain to tell us when we are hungry. Recent experimental work also shows an association between hunger pangs and glucose utilization, but scientists have not as yet been able to describe the entire process in detail.

This normal fluctuation in blood-sugar level and the occurrence of hunger pangs make an obese person just as hungry as a thin one.

If eating is postponed after the brain and stomach have sent out their signals, sugar levels fall still further. It is not at all unusual for blood-sugar level to drop below normal; and it is not difficult to *make* it drop below normal simply by not eating for an extended period of time.

Even in the rare cases where true or reactive hypoglycemia does occur, legitimate specialists in the field are unlikely to consider it a disease as such. Rather, they tend to regard it as a symptom. And much as a runny nose may be a symptom of a cold or an allergic reaction or some other condition, so does true hypoglycemia indicate that something in the body's mechanism is not working correctly. There are various possibilities, but, most commonly, continued low blood-sugar levels are caused by tumors in the pancreas that lead to an overproduction of insulin.

Popular "wisdom" has decreed that too much sugar in the diet (particularly refined sugar, of course) also stimulates the pancreas to produce too much insulin, thus leading to lowered blood sugar. This is unadulterated hogwash and contrary to the known facts of sugar metabolism.

Nevertheless, we occasionally encounter the fashionable theory that hypoglycemia is responsible for an amazing amount of antisocial behavior. Many misconceptions about this nondisease prompted the following joint public statement in 1973 by the American Diabetes Association, the Endocrine Society, and the American Medical Association:

"When [hypoglycemia] occurs, it is often attended by symptoms of sweating, shakiness, trembling, anxiety, fast heart action, headache, hunger sensations, brief feelings of weakness, and, occasionally, seizures and coma. However, the majority of people with these kinds of symptoms do not have hypoglycemia; a great many patients with anxiety reactions present similar symptoms. Furthermore, there is no good evidence that hypoglycemia causes depression, chronic fatigue, allergies, nervous breakdowns, alcoholism, juvenile delinquency, childhood behavior problems, drug addiction, or inadequate sexual performance. . . ."

However convenient a crutch hypoglycemia may provide, the fact is that it is simply not a legitimate diagnosis for the vast majority of the population.

TOOTH DECAY

Sugar can indeed contribute to dental caries. What few people understand, however, is that the sticky sugars eaten between meals do the major damage. Sugar consumed with meals or in liquids does appreciably less harm, or no harm, to the teeth. Further, the *amount* of sugar in a food appears to be less important in the development of dental caries than the frequency of eating and the length of time the sugar remains in contact with the teeth. Other carbohydrates, such as starch, also contribute to tooth decay because much of the starch is rapidly converted to glucose by the saliva in the mouth.

Briefly, what happens is this: A great many bacteria normally inhabit the mouth (and, TV commercials aside, mouthwashes have little effect on their survival rate). These bacteria manufacture weak organic acids from sugar and other carbohydrates. The bacteria multiply and form a plaque on the teeth. The organic acids they make can erode tooth enamel and thus lead to cavities. It should be readily apparent that the longer a carbohydrate remains in contact with the teeth, the longer the production of these destructive acids.

This concept has been illustrated by the well-known Vipeholm Study, an extensive project conducted carefully many years ago at an institute in Sweden over a period of five years. The results, supported by a considerable amount of additional research by other scientists, may be summed up this way:

- Eliminating all table sugar from the diet did not prevent cavities.
- Sugar consumed at mealtime in amounts that were double that of the average population had no appreciable effect on cavity development. (That is, the number of cavities differed very little from those in subjects receiving only an average amount of sugar, or no sugar at all.)
- Increased frequency of brushing produced fewer cavities than infrequent brushing by subjects consuming identical diets.
- High amounts of sugar consumed in beverages with meals made a barely perceptible increase in the development of cavities.
- Sugar consumed in chocolate caused increases in dental caries that were intermediate, as compared with sticky candy and sweet beverages. (Interestingly, more recent studies indicate that chocolate may actually have an *inhibiting* effect on dental caries.)
- The stickiness of a sweet food consumed between meals is the single greatest contributor to tooth decay. Even though the food may be relatively less sweet than many nonsticky items, the very sticky ones are those that remain in longest contact with the teeth. Substances like sweet toffees can cause a great amount of damage if they are not promptly brushed away.

In other words, the total amount of sugar consumed is not the critical factor in determining the amount of tooth decay. *Exposure time* is what we need to be concerned with.

205

Sugars consumed at mealtime tend to be cleansed away by the other foods eaten and drunk with the meal. And sugars in beverages are quickly washed away.

Don't be misled that dental problems can be avoided by replacing table sugar with good old "natural" honey or dried fruits. Bacteria aren't the least bit particular about the kinds of sugar they feed on; they're just as fond of honey and fruit sugar as they are of the refined white stuff in the sugar bowl. (And foods such as raisins nestling among the teeth can provide hours of tasty fare for bacteria.) Again, this fact has been borne out by a number of studies. Even in the Vipeholm Study, the highest cavity group consisted of subjects who ate sweet clinging toffees between meals—and those toffees actually contained more *lactose* (milk sugar) than sucrose.

Further, don't let anyone convince you that special health foods can prevent tooth decay. Favorite products promoted for that purpose are bone meal and dolomite, both of which are essentially useless. The minerals they contain are easily available in any halfway balanced diet. But minerals in any form, except for fluoride, do not prevent cavities resulting from plaque.

Tooth decay can be minimized—or, for a lucky few, even prevented—by good dental care. That means correct, thorough, frequent brushing and regular dental checkups. Fluoridation programs give an even greater boost to good dental health. Unlike the groundless recommendations to cut back sugar consumption as a means of controlling tooth decay, our recommendation for fluoridated water *does* have a great deal of scientific evidence on which to rest.

By 1970, at least fourteen separate studies had been conducted on the use of fluoridated water over a period of ten years or more, and hundreds of other studies for shorter periods of time. The results are very impressive. For example, a fifteen-year study in Grand Rapids, Michigan, of children using fluoridated water from birth showed 50–63 percent less tooth decay than among their counterparts in nonfluoridated areas. Ten years after fluoridation, six-to-nine-year-old children in Newburgh,

New York, were experiencing 58 percent less tooth decay than the same age group in nearby, nonfluoridated Kingston, New York. Older children who received fluoridated water for only a few years showed 41 percent less decay.

In lieu of total fluoridation, there are other options. The National Institute of Dental Research recently sponsored a school-based fluoride-mouth-rinsing program. The results, released in 1978, noted a reduction in dental caries of 35 percent for the 75,-000 children included in the study. If such a program were put into effect nationally, scientists estimate that a mere fifty cents per student per year could save a total of several billion dollars annually in dental costs.

Even the cost of fluoridating the public water supply is minimal. The benefits are enormous. Yet, nationwide, a vast number of communities are forced to forego these benefits.

Fluoridation of the water supply does not pose any type of health hazard, but misinformation has led to a groundless fear of adding "chemicals" to the water, and people argue that they should have a choice, rather than be forced to consume fluoridated water.

HEART DISEASE

The most vigorously publicized proposal that sugar is a causative factor in heart disease is that of an English physician, Dr. John Yudkin, but just how he managed to arrive at that theory is perplexing. His major study in "support" of his hypothesis was comprised of exactly twenty persons, and careful analysis of the data reveals that these heart patients consumed about as much sugar as did their fellow countrymen. Yet Yudkin somehow drew the mystifying conclusion that sugar is bad for the heart.

Invalid as it might be, the theory provided meaty material for the news media. Headlines and TV programs again shouted their warnings, and the American public was left with still one more threat to worry about needlessly. When other scientists set out to duplicate Yudkin's findings, they could not. Some studies even found that heart patients consumed *less* sugar than average.

None of this, of course, attracted anywhere near the publicity of Yudkin's original statements. After all, what *doesn't* happen is not very exciting news.

A quick look at some simple statistics will illustrate why the sugar-heart disease theory makes so little sense. If the relationship were positive, then countries with high sugar consumption should have a higher rate of heart disease. This is not necessarily the case. Very high-sugar-consumption countries such as Venezuela, Cuba, the Honduras, Costa Rica, and others have a rather low incidence of heart disease. We have already noted that sugar consumption in the United States has remained almost constant during the past fifty years; yet the incidence of heart disease has risen considerably.

When asked their opinions about a sugar-heart association, informed scientists almost unanimously echo such observations as that expressed by Dr. Francisco Grande, formerly professor of physiological hygiene at the University of Minnesota's School of Public Health. After an extensive review of all available literature on the subject, Grande asserted: "The weight of evidence seems to be against any direct association between high sucrose intake and the development of coronary heart disease."

LEARNING DISABILITIES

In this case, there simply aren't even any scientific studies to refute. We hear a great deal about sugar allegedly creating learning difficulties, but what is being circulated is a combination of testimonials, opinion, and conjecture. Indeed, *science* indicates that the very opposite may be true. Without ample supplies of blood glucose, the brain simply cannot function properly. This is not to imply that one *must* consume some sugar. Starch is also a source of blood glucose.

This and the following topic will be discussed further in chapter 9 on nutrition and behavior.

HYPERKINESIS

Now that research has acquitted food additives as the major cause of hyperactivity (hyperkinesis) in children, a different dietary culprit has been called up: As you might expect, it's sugar. Evidence "linking" sugar and hyperactivity is strictly anecdotal. For instance, the argument has been used that children are more restless than usual in school on the day after Halloween. While it has been a year or two since we went trick-or-treating, we do remember that there was more to that delightful holiday than just eating candy. If children seem distracted on November 1, it seems reasonable to suggest that the excitement and adventure of the previous evening are more likely responsible for their behavior than what they had to eat.

CONSTIPATION

Here again we encounter an unfounded charge. When sugars, or any sweets, are consumed as part of a balanced diet, there is no reason whatever to suspect they cause constipation. When eaten in *excessive* amounts, however, sugar products sometimes replace needed fiber in the diet. Insufficient dietary fiber could very well contribute to elimination difficulties. But sugar itself is not at fault.

A NUTRIENT DANGER?

There is nothing in the medical or other scientific literature to indicate that sugar uniquely increases our requirements for certain nutrients. Yet repeatedly we come across such blarney, as in Naura Hayden's *Everything You've Always Wanted to Know About Energy But Were Too Weak to Ask*: "Sugar, to be metabolized, must burn up all the B vites [Haydenese for "vitamins"] in your system in the metabolic process." Hayden's credentials, if such exist, go unmentioned; her chief claim to fame is apparently her acquaintance with a few big names in Hollywood who disapprove of sugar. One fact is certain: She is no student of nutrition or any other science. What she is presenting is a distortion of the well-known scientific fact that requirements for certain B vitamins increase with a greater intake of carbohydrates. B vitamins are needed for the metabolism of carbohydrates but are not "burned up" during sugar metabolism. It is true that refined sugars do not contain any of the B vitamins. But a varied, well-balanced diet normally contains sufficient B vitamins to meet nutritional requirements.

When sugar products are consumed *in place of* other needed nutrients, deficiencies can certainly occur. But here again, it is not sugar that fosters the damage; it is the simple absence of one or more components of a balanced diet. This is precisely the same principle involved in the allegation that sugar is found chiefly in something called "junk food."

The question is: What exactly *is* junk food? By definition, junk is valueless refuse, implying that junk food must be something retrieved from the garbage can. But perhaps we are being a bit frivolous. While no one seems able to define precisely the meaning of the term, it is generally assumed that "junk food" is anything edible that is high in sugar, fat, and calories. The term is, however, a misnomer. All foods—again, by definition—contain some nutrients. A lopsided combination of foods can result in a *junk diet,* but no single food can be considered junk unless it crowds out of the diet other foods necessary for good nutrition. Thus, a diet consisting chiefly of candy bars and carmel corn may be considered a junk diet. A diet consisting chiefly of carrots and cream cheese may also be considered a junk diet. It is true, however, that the *former* junk diet is more common among children, who often fill up on these foods and then are unable to eat food served to them at mealtime.

Similarly, the charge that sugar is "full of empty calories" is plain silly. As mentioned earlier, all calories are full calories, full of energy. A calorie is a measurement of heat energy, and one calorie is one unit of energy, regardless of its source. As long as the Recommended Dietary Allowance is being met for all nutrients, there is no harm whatever in using snack foods to fulfill additional calorie requirements. If you have a weight problem, you won't have room for very many of these "extras"; if you are on a reducing diet, chances are you will temporarily have to do without any at all, but that doesn't mean eliminating all sugar. (And if you have high blood pressure, you should keep salty snacks to a bare minimum.)

Candy and other sweets aren't intended to serve the same purpose in the diet as other foods, but this doesn't mean they are totally devoid of nutrients either. In addition to energy-giving sugar, sweets frequently contain milk, eggs, nuts, or dried fruits and offer small amounts of all the nutrients present in those excellent foods. Chocolate provides riboflavin, calcium, and iron. Nuts in candies supply protein, calcium, iron, and several B vitamins.

Let's not minimize the psychological value of sweet treats as well. Candy has been held in favor for some 4,000 years.

SUGAR ''ADDICTION''

Many people think that if a child never eats sugar or sugar products, he will never get into "the habit" of enjoying them. Sugar is decidedly not a food item that anyone has to "learn" to like. Tartar steak, turnip greens, tea, and tabasco sauce represent but a fraction of the many items that are usually enjoyed only after acquiring a taste for them (which many people never do). But studies reveal that day-old infants sampling their first taste of sugar water invariably indicate a preference for it over plain water.

Yet some peculiar opinions have evolved. Dr. David Reuben, in his book *Everything You Always Wanted to Know About Nutrition*, devotes an entire chapter to "cocainelike" sugar—with its implicit suggestion that anyone reckless enough to partake of the evil sweetness will be doomed to a life of misery. We can only guess where Reuben acquired much of his statistical misinformation, but we suspect that he must have been doing a certain amount of guessing. He has attempted to convince his readers that per capita sugar consumption in the United States ranges between 150 and 175 pounds per year. That's just about 50 to 75 percent more than the plus-or-minus average of 100 annual pounds, disappearance data from USDA.

Physiologically, the human body requires a regular intake of carbohydrates, though not necessarily in the form of sugar. But psychologically, sugar is "addictive" only in the sense that people tend to consume foods they enjoy—and, for most people, sugar contributes to that enjoyment.

The Presweetened Cereal Controversy

Modern-day cereal magnates have come under a new kind of attack. At every turn, parents are warned of the "hazards" of presweetened cereals. One waggish naturalist, in a cute attempt to illustrate his antisugar argument, fed a single rat a presweetened cereal while offering one additional rat only the pulverized cereal box. The box-eating rat was the only one expected to thrive, but, as you might guess, the results of this "study" were inconclusive.

"START THE DAY WITH A GOOD BREAKFAST"

Before we jump into the middle of the presweetened vs. postsweetened controversy, let's first take a look at the importance of cereal itself.

Nutritionists almost unanimously agree that breakfast should provide at least one-quarter of the day's Recommended Dietary Allowances. Almost all ready-to-eat cereals, presweetened or otherwise, are fortified at that level with seven major nutrients: vitamins A, C, B_6, thiamine, riboflavin, niacin, and folic acid. Other vitamins and minerals are usually present in lesser amounts. By law, this information must be included on the package label. A careful check will readily inform you that a serving of fortified cereal, with the addition of milk, does indeed provide the basis for a healthful, nutritious breakfast for children and adults alike. Add citrus fruit or juice, or some other vitamin C-rich fruit, and a piece of toast or a muffin, and you have it made.

The question occasionally arises whether such cereals really replace a hearty American breakfast of bacon, eggs, and toast. The answer is no. The taste and texture of bacon and eggs are uniquely bacon and eggs. You should know, however, that non-cereal breakfasts invariably contain much more fat and are much lower in vitamin and iron content. If you and your family enjoy bacon and eggs, there is no reason not to serve them occasionally, but fortified cereals generally provide superior nutrition.

Parents of school-age children are well aware that these cereals are also a convenient aid in surviving the morning household rush. Still, there are also those parents who, feeling somewhat guilty about serving a hurry-up menu of cereal, milk, and juice, instead decide to substitute hot oatmeal for that fortified cereal. Or they may feel that only an "all-natural" cereal like granola is acceptable. Again, check those labels! You may be surprised to find that neither product approaches the nutrient levels of most ready-to-eats, and they probably have more calories.

SUGAR, SUGAR, EVERYWHERE

For generations, most people have sprinkled sugar over their cereal before eating it. In an effort to tempt young palates into eating a nutritious breakfast, cereal manufacturers some years ago began developing new kinds of cereal with the sugar already on it. Most children have indeed found at least some of the pre-sweetened varieties to be more interesting and tasty than the regular kinds. But their parents are concerned about "all that sugar." Because sugar is occasionally listed as the first ingredient on the package, indicating that its quantity is greater than any other ingredient, many have the distorted impression that what they are really eating is a gob of sugar with a little dash of cereal in it. That is far from the real picture.

To begin with, an average one-ounce serving of presweetened cereal contains about 11 grams of sugar. When you compare that with the 17 grams of sugar in a medium-sized apple, for instance, the amount doesn't seem quite so horrendous.

Second, research demonstrates that children (and adults) actually consume *less* sugar at breakfast when they eat it in the form of presweetened cereal. A recent study conducted with more than a thousand children in nine cities compared the quantity of sugar in presweetened cereals with that in regular varieties that had been sweetened from the sugar bowl. In each comparison, total available sugar was greater in the servings of regular cereal to which children added their own sugar. (To be fair, we should point out that some of the sugar-bowl sugar occasionally sinks to the bottom of the cereal dish and may be thrown out along with the leftover milk.)

Succumbing to consumer pressure, some of the cereal companies have apparently exerted a concentrated effort to see that a few newer brands do not give the impression that they are mostly sugar. Such products as Frosted Rice, Honeycombs, and Wheat Chex, for instance, listed sugar as the second ingredient. Kellogg's new Raisins, Rice and Rye has sugar as only its fourth ingredient. A quick glance will tell you that such old standbys as Cornflakes and Cheerios—which few would consider a presweetened product—nevertheless also contain a small amount of sugar.

While you are comparing labels, you should also note that most ready-to-eat cereals contain approximately the same number of calories. The slight variations are completely independent of whether or not they have been presweetened. Furthermore, there is no indication that cereal eaten *with milk* contributes to dental caries. A study was conducted in a boarding school in Wisconsin with 145 subjects from age 13 to 18 to investigate the correlation between ready-to-eat cereals and dental caries. The study concluded no statistically significant difference between the incidence of dental caries among cereal eaters and that among noncereal eaters, or between the users of presweetened and non-presweetened cereals. There have been perhaps a dozen similar studies, some with far larger numbers of children, and the results are all the same.

The bottom line of the cereal controversy is that you may safely eat whatever kind of cereal appeals to you. We'll be the first

to admit that some of the so-called "children's" cereals often
have strange flavors (even to children). But taste and nutrient
content should govern your choice, rather than any miscon-
ceived concern about sugar.

Conclusions

The results of studies conducted by a group of impartial scientists for the Food and Drug Administration, released in 1977,
have indicated that "there is no clear evidence in the available
information on sucrose that demonstrates a hazard to the public
when used at the levels that are now current and in the manner
now practiced."

Just because sugar tastes good doesn't mean it is bad for you.
Sugar is a first-rate source of energy. Relax and enjoy moderate
amounts, if that is your pleasure.

CHAPTER 8

Vitamins: If a Little Is Good, More Must Be Better

IS EMOTIONAL STRESS MAKING YOUR LIFE miserable? Pop a few pills of vitamin C. Sex life growing stale? Worried about air pollution? A few hundred units of vitamin E is the remedy. So go the claims of the enthusiasts who fancy that health and happiness can be purchased in little bottles. Don't you believe it!

The Need for Nutrients

The human body is an extremely complex machine. To function efficiently, it requires the presence of some fifty different nutrients, which continually interact in an intricate series of chemical reactions. The *absence* of any single essential nutrient over a period of time will produce a deficiency disease. This does not mean that *excessive* amounts of the same nutrient will either pre-

216

vent or cure disease. The body requires specific amounts; it has no use for excesses.

As an extremely simplified illustration, suppose that we are attempting to produce a small flask of water in a laboratory. Almost everyone is aware that water is composed of hydrogen and oxygen in a ratio of two to one (H_2O). If we add additional hydrogen to the chemical reaction to make water, we do not get more water unless additional oxygen is also added. And once we have enough water to fill the flask, no amount of hydrogen or oxygen will put additional water into that flask.

The same is true of the human body. "Leftover" nutrients are either excreted as waste or stored in the body, occasionally reaching dangerously high levels. No one nutrient performs a single function, and no nutrient performs *any* function without the aid of other substances that are specifically required for that function.

We have long been told, for instance, that vitamin A is "good for the eyes." It is, although it is important for other reasons as well, but by itself it cannot benefit the eyes or any other part of the body. But, confining ourselves for the moment to the eyes, vitamin A deficiency over a period of time leads to obstructed tear ducts and impaired vision in dim light (so-called "night blindness"). Severe deficiency leads to total blindness, a condition not uncommon in parts of Asia and the Middle East. Vitamin A supplements will correct a vitamin A deficiency, but they will not prevent any other types of blindness from occurring; nor will they cure blindness or other visual disorders such as nearsightedness, astigmatism, or cataracts, which are not caused by a lack of vitamin A. Similarly, because it was known that a severe deficiency of vitamin A could cause skin lesions, supplements were at one time prescribed to "cure" certain skin conditions such as acne; but there is little evidence of their effectiveness (and a great deal of evidence that high doses can prove toxic).

TOO MUCH OF A GOOD THING

While it is important to understand that very large amounts (megadoses) of vitamin A are useless for anyone not suffering from vitamin A deficiency, it is *vital* to understand that these same megadoses can be exceedingly dangerous. A small serving of carrots will supply the average person with enough vitamin A for two days. What the body doesn't use, it stores in the liver. For this reason, animal liver is an excellent source of that vitamin. Eskimos learned long ago to avoid eating polar-bear liver, even though they did not know the reason that it caused death was its extremely high vitamin A content: about one million international units (IU) in three ounces, compared to a Recommended Dietary Allowance of 4,000 IU for females and 5,000 IU for males. (In other words, a small serving of polar-bear liver contains 200 to 250 times the RDA.)

Between 1960 and 1964, approximately twenty children in New York died from hypervitaminosis A because their mothers, marching to the "more is better" tune, doubled the recommended dosage of vitamin supplements, giving each child two capsules daily in addition to the more than adequate amounts they were already receiving from the milk, butter or margarine, and vegetables in their diet.

Vitamin A and vitamin D are of particular concern because even in doses which are commonly purchased at pharmacies or health-food stores, supplements can be harmful. Too much of *any* nutrient can be disastrous. Yet small health-food stores and major pharmaceutical houses alike are marketing supernutrition, and the American public is being continually treated to a substantial helping of myth along with their dietary supplements.

THE MODERN ''MEDICINE MEN''

The public is gullible. Their fears aroused by inconclusive research studies and spurred on by slanted media stories, people are eager to try almost anything to forestall or cure cancer, arthritis, obesity, heart disease, diabetes, headache, nervousness, constipation, aging, baldness, and rundownitis. They are willing to spend billions of dollars every year for vitamins, minerals, and "wonder" substances that for the most part are virtually useless. Nutrition misinformation and public fear have coupled to produce a new breed of quack whose slogan is, "If a little is good, a great deal must be better." The dosages recommended are usually several times—or even several hundred times—more than any one person's body could possibly use during the course of a day. If the nutrient is water soluble, most of it usually passes on through to nurture whatever forms of life may inhabit the local sewage system; if the nutrient is not soluble in water, it is stored in the body, where it may eventually accumulate to toxic levels and produce untold misery.

Although we have just used the singular form of the word nutrient, few health faddists are content to limit themselves to a mere one or two supplemental nutrients. Each one is usually purported to prevent or cure a long and diverse list of symptoms, but the most avid adherents are taking no chances! Just to be sure, they assemble an entire conglomeration of daily dietary supplements. Health-food stores even sell compartmented pill containers, but the most devout of the pill lovers find fishermen's tackleboxes more spacious for housing their supplies (à la Adelle Davis). It may sound like a joke, but it isn't.

The supplement pushers are evidently achieving considerable success. Several national surveys during the past few years reveal that approximately 75 percent of the adult population thinks that extra vitamins promote extra pep and energy, and lead to better health generally. Whether due to a lack of basic health education, or because the surge of propaganda has eventually overpowered their common sense, too few people seem to be aware of the saturation levels for vitamins or other nutrients—the point beyond which excessive amounts cannot be utilized. Further, not nearly enough people seem to understand that *all* nutrients are readily available from the food in a balanced diet. The only exceptions here are iron, which is poorly absorbed and occasionally insufficient, particularly in the diets of women of childbearing age; and fluoride, unless one has access to fluoridated water. Other than that, as we saw in chapter 2, nutrient deficiencies are uncommon in most areas of the United States. In poverty areas, nutrition is often a serious problem, but what the inhabitants there need is *food*, not supplements. In affluent societies, the problem is just the opposite. Too much food is consumed, and obesity results.

"Trace nutrient" has lately become the catch phrase, as in, "This valuable trace element may be lacking in your diet!" The truth is that trace elements are almost *never* lacking in any diet based on the Basic Four Food Groups. As the name implies, trace elements are required in such minute amounts that unless a specific metabolic disturbance is present, deficiency is next to impossible to achieve, even when the daily fare is somewhat lacking in optimal balance.

A danger just as serious as too few nutrients is the eventual toxic effect of too many. The human body is simply not equipped to handle on a daily basis the amount of vitamin C equivalent to an entire carload of oranges or the vitamin A from a carload of carrots. As with salt, a minimal amount is necessary to maintain life; too much can be lethal. In this country, the toxic effects of excess doses of vitamins (particularly the fat-soluble ones) are now more frequently seen by doctors than the classical vitamin deficiency diseases such as scurvy, pellagra, and beriberi.

THE VITAMIN DOCTORS

What is even more disturbing than the fallacies bandied about by unprofessional health-food faddists is the evolution of a new breed of physicians who prescribe massive doses of vitamins and other nutrient supplements. For example, a New York City psychiatrist, Dr. Henry Newbold, advocates niacin as a weapon against heart disease—in amounts up to 150 times the Recommended Dietary Allowance.

Prescriptions may be for any specific condition, or simply to promote a general sense of well-being, but particular attention is currently focused on a relatively new field known as orthomolecular psychiatry. Its founders, Dr. Abram Hoffer and Dr. Humphry Osmond, claim that megadosing in specific combinations can effectively treat—and sometimes cure—schizophrenia, alcoholism, drug addition, hyperactivity in children, and other forms of psychological disturbances.

Psychiatrists and other physicians have long been aware of the association between certain physical conditions and psychological disorders; they are just as aware that there are as yet many unopened doors. But indiscriminate megadosing on a long-term basis is simply not a safe method of treatment for either psychiatric disorders or any other medical problem. In a *Journal of the American Medical Association* editorial (August 11, 1975), Dr. Philip L. White, director of the AMA's Department of Food and Nutrition, states: "If there were some objective evidence that megavitamin therapy or orthomolecular psychiatry produced beneficial results, one would then use the rule of reason in evaluating the risk-benefit ratio. For the present, we can only conclude that there is no benefit to massive daily doses of the vitamins and that only one aspect can be evaluated, namely, the risk."

THE NEED FOR BALANCE

A further hidden danger of megadosing is the effect that too much of a given nutrient may have on other nutrients or compounds in the body, and the body chemistry as a whole. As mentioned earlier in this book, bran—one of the so-called "wonder foods"—in large daily amounts can bind with iron in the body and carry it right on through, without it being absorbed. Similarly, Popeye would have been astonished to learn that although his beloved spinach does indeed contain a large amount of iron, the oxalates also present in that vegetable keep a considerable amount of it in a form that cannot be utilized by the body. All nutrients interact in the body in a very complex fashion. When one or more of them is disproportionately high, it may affect certain of the others.

Scientists have already spent a great many years determining what nutrients, in what quantities, people need for good health. While future research may reveal that minor adjustments are indicated, it is illogical to assume that after decades of study by countless nutritional experts, the results are meaningless.

Vitamins and minerals in proper amounts are essential for good health; beyond that they are not miracle potions. They will neither cure nor prevent anything other than a deficiency of that particular vitamin or mineral. And when we speak of deficiency, we are not alluding to a self-diagnosed deficiency. We mean a *medically* diagnosed deficiency, usually established by laboratory testing. The special danger of self-prescription is the possibility—a rather frequent one—that you may be "treating" the wrong condition. The person who prescribes for himself massive doses of vitamin C to overcome recurring symptoms of the common cold may actually be suffering from a severe sinus condition or allergic reaction; or even a lung disorder, which, left untreated, will gradually worsen.

Occasionally a metabolic defect will prevent the body from utilizing a nutrient, even though it is present in sufficient amounts in the diet. A classic example is pernicious anemia, an illness caused by the inability to absorb vitamin B_{12}. Here, some form of B_{12} supplementation by injection is necessary. An oral supplement of B_{12} would not correct the deficiency, because it would not be metabolized. And this does not mean, contrary to many vitamin ads, that B_{12} supplements will prevent the condition from occurring in the first place.

It is worthwhile noting here that B_{12} is found only in foods of animal origin. Strict vegetarians—that is, those whose diets contain no milk, eggs, butter, or other animal products—do require a B_{12} supplement. But as an example of how small are the needed amounts (3 micrograms per day),* Hindus living in India and consuming no animal products whatever do not take B_{12} supplements and do not develop a vitamin B_{12} deficiency. The reason is that they ingest enough B_{12} from the insect parts that are an in-

---

* A microgram is one-millionth of a gram.

advertent contaminant of the other foods they eat. Studies show, however, that Hindus emigrating to England, where the food is cleaner, do develop a B_{12} deficiency.

A botanist at Washington University in St. Louis claims that B_{12} also occurs naturally in rainwater. Perhaps this indicates that regularly standing in the rain for ten minutes or so with one's mouth open would eliminate the need for other sources of this vitamin, but we do not advise it. More likely, the rain water barrel had a few bugs in it, and these little animals provided the vitamin B_{12}.

Individuals following weight-reducing diets often feel a need to take extra vitamins to make up for those that are not being eaten; indeed, some regimens even include supplements as part of the diet. A good reducing diet should be well balanced to supply adequate amounts of nutrients. However, even on a well-planned reducing diet, it can be difficult to meet all of your needs for nutrients if you are consuming relatively few calories. This is one of the few situations where a low-dose multivitamin/mineral supplement (one that supplies less or certainly no more than 100 percent of the U.S. Recommended Daily Allowance of any nutrient) may be useful. If you are going to be on a diet that allows less than 1,500 calories per day for a substantial length of time, you may want to check with your doctor to see if a low-dose supplement might be advisable. But, like everyone else, dieters don't need vitamins or minerals in amounts greater than the recommended allowances. In fact, experiments with laboratory animals have demonstrated that excessive amounts of vitamins actually act as an appetite stimulant. While we don't know if the same is true for humans, it does suggest that dieters have even more reason than other people to avoid excess supplements.

Unneeded supplements upset the nutrient balance. Scientists know that the possibilities of adverse reactions are so far-reaching that many are yet to be uncovered.

WONDER FOODS

The preoccupation with vitamins has led to a revival of a number of food items that folklore has endowed with magical properties. In the interest of progress—and steadily ringing cash registers—a few newcomers have joined the ranks. The discerning palate may assert that "food" is a euphemistic term for such substances as alfalfa, bee pollen, ginseng root, and apple-cider vinegar. Although we do refer to them as foods since they *are* edible, bear in mind that that is perhaps the nicest thing we can say about many of these so-called "wonder" products.

There is nothing wondrous about any of them except their prices and the claims for their benefits. There is no single specific food, or limited combination of specific foods, that is mandatory for good health or that will prevent disease. Brewer's yeast, for example, is indeed rich in B vitamins and protein; so are a great many other foods. There is simply no reason to add such an unpalatable substance to your diet, unless by some remote chance you happen to positively enjoy it.

LEGISLATION

Any thinking person will be quick to question why, if megadosing is so potentially harmful, the marketing of vitamins and similar products is not regulated by law. The Food and Drug Administration has indeed attempted to curb over-the-counter megavitamin sales, but its efforts have so far met with little success. The legal question is sticky, since dietary supplements are technically neither foods nor drugs. That issue has been the subject of more than one lawsuit against the FDA, and extensive letter-writing campaigns by the health-food industry have managed to squelch most official intervention. (There are a few exceptions: Liquid protein diets, for example, must now carry a warning label.)

As we mentioned earlier, product labels cannot legally include false or unsubstantiated claims; but pamphlets, books, and speeches about them can, and do—prolifically.

We're totally in favor of freedom of the press and freedom of speech. What is unfortunate is that the misguided use of either can create unrealistic demands and pressures. The official legislative position at present seems to be that vitamin and mineral supplements, taken in correct amounts, are no more dangerous than aspirin; that it is only their *misuse* that is potentially harmful. Tragically, as more and more people are heeding the scientifically unsupported propaganda of health-food merchants and so-called health books, misuse of dietary supplements is growing rampant.

A fine line separates precisely what constitutes "false and misleading advertising" and what does not. Thus, supplement ads are very carefully and cleverly written, and every syllable scrutinized by bright corporate attorneys. Often the brand names themselves are very appealing. Zoom, Force, Preventron (offering "high-potency protection"), Pep Tabs, Vita-Go, and Master Formula all sound like potions no one should be without. Another, More, boasts sixty-four different ingredients in a "natural food base" that includes black molasses powder and fish-liver oil, typical of most of the multiingredient compounds. The accompanying copy implies that the product is a must for good health, but it does not specifically state so; and thus there is nothing illegal in its advertisements.

For the past-middle-age individual, there are multi-compounds like Ger-E-Mates and Geri-Max; for children, Super Child and Child Love. Other preparations appeal to women on the Pill, or purport to be specifically designed for athletes or menopause or pregnancy or the "active woman." Another, with the enticing name Gerovital and aimed at the middle-aged and elderly, has as its active ingredient procaine, an anesthetic derivative of novocaine. It is illegal in the United States at the moment—but the pressure is on.

Throughout the rest of the chapter, we will examine a few of the claims noted in our perusal of ads for such products as herbal diuretics, alfalfa tablets, "multiminerals," acidophilus capsules, hair-care vitamins, bran tablets, stress formulas, grapefruit pills, desiccated liver tablets, beef-spleen extract, and garlic-oil capsules. (Not to worry: The latter "dissolves in your stomach, not in your mouth.")

If you have an ailment, someone has a "nutritious" pill for it.

Vitamins

"How much of your vitamin C gets lost on the way to the table?" There is certainly nothing illegal in leading off an advertisement with that question. But it is surely designed to frighten the consumer into running to the store for some vitamin C tablets. True, C is one of the more fragile vitamins, and it is partially destroyed by prolonged storage and exposure to air. But even a minimum of common-sense food care allows the average person easily to obtain his RDA by consuming one serving of a vitamin C-rich food daily.

"Your body functions demand extra amounts of 'B' daily to help cope with stress and tension."

"Packaged sunshine," Vitamins A and D, "keep a high immune response in your system to protect you against environmental stress."

"Golden E-Oil for dry, aging, wrinkly skin."

A supercompound for the elderly offers "built-in digestive power" with its "therapeutic nutritional protection against daily stress."

The ads run on and on with their glowing promises. But because most of us have learned to be at least a little skeptical about advertising, what is even more disturbing are the pamphlets, leaflets, and brochures freely distributed by health-food stores and wholesalers. They cover a wide assortment of topics and tend to express the most outlandish theories and hypotheses as pure fact. The uninformed consumer may understandably be frightened at reading, for instance, that in an aging body or one subjected to extreme stress, the stomach does not produce enough hydrochloric acid and enzymes to digest food properly, thus leading to "malnutrition" and the need for extra vitamins. It is not unlikely that such a consumer will rush to buy not only a supervitamin formula, but one that also contains hydrochloric acid and plenty of enzymes.

The sad fact is that too low a secretion of hydrochloric acid (hypochlorhydria), when it exists at all, is almost always a symptom of some relatively serious medical condition meriting the immediate attention of a physician.* Further, ingested enzymes are totally useless since they are destroyed in the stomach by that same hydrochloric acid that either accompanies them in the preparations, or is already present in the stomach. The situation would be absurd if it were less reprehensible. Yet it is typical of the kind of malarkey continually foisted on the public and not subject to legal restriction.

No one has to look very far to encounter such vitamin hogwash as the following:

- that vitamin A will prevent some cancers, improve the skin, and cure learning disabilities;
- that vitamin B_1 (thiamine) functions as an antidepressant and reduces cravings for certain drugs;
- that vitamin B_2 (riboflavin) will overcome stress;
- that vitamin B_3 (niacin) stabilizes manic-depressive psychosis, relieves schizophrenia, and improves circulation in the elderly;
- that vitamin B_5 (pantothenic acid) restores color to gray hair (it does, in rats);
- that vitamin B_6 (pyridoxine) overcomes fatigue, anxiety, and depression, and relieves Parkinson's disease. (It does not, and, paradoxically, an excess of B_6 can block the effectiveness of certain drugs like L-dopa, often used in the treatment of this disease.);
- that vitamin B_{12} can relieve neuritis, neuralgia, and psoriasis, and is a hangover remedy of long standing;

* Hypochlorhydria is also sometimes present in certain types of psychosis and neurosis.

227

- that vitamin C (ascorbic acid) prevents colds, cures cancer, relieves back pain, and lowers cholesterol. (As Dr. Linus Pauling's favorite vitamin, he recommends it for almost everything.);
- that vitamin D promotes general well-being;
- that vitamin E will do almost anything: overcome impotence, promote fertility, prevent aging, promote healthy skin, aid in weight reduction, prevent miscarriage, minimize birth deformities, dissolve blood clots; that it will prevent and treat high blood pressure, kidney disease, rheumatic fever, most forms of heart disease and varicose veins; that external application helps wounds and burns to heal without scars; and that taken from an early age, it will prevent senility and stroke;
- that biotin (a member of the B complex but also sometimes known as vitamin H, for some mysterious reason) aids scalp problems, thinning hair, and baldness;
- that folic acid (also belonging to the B complex) cures nervous disorders and prevents leukemia.

Additional claims are often made that the use of contraceptive pills requires an additional vitamin intake. While it is indeed true that women on the "Pill" should take extra care in achieving a balanced diet, there is no need for vitamin supplements unless a specific deficiency has been diagnosed. Similarly, supplemental B vitamins are often touted as essential for those consuming alcoholic beverages. This, too, is nonsense. Chronic alcoholics are frequently deficient in thiamine; they are also frequently deficient in a number of other nutrients. The deficiencies are caused primarily by the alcoholic's tendency not to eat a balanced diet. No amount of thiamine or B complex will cure alcoholism, nor will it prevent the malnutrition that results in those who habitually substitute drinking for eating.

The list of proclamations is endless, but space permits only the above representative sampling. "Try-anything" customers could be kept busy for years experimenting with different combinations.

FROM TOO LITTLE TO TOO MUCH

What the ads, booklets, flyers, and posters usually don't tell you about are the hazardous, sometimes lethal, effects of overdosing, or hypervitaminosis. The Food and Drug Administration has widely reported the story of a teenage girl who was being prepared for surgery for a brain tumor when it was discovered that her symptoms actually resulted from the massive amounts of vitamin A in her body. In other cases, vitamin A toxicity has also led to false diagnoses of meningitis.

Tragedy is not always prevented, however. A few years ago a mother in Maine alleged she had given her young daughter large doses of vitamin A after reading Adelle Davis' recommendations in *Let's Have Healthy Children* (Harcourt Brace Jovanovich, 1972). As a result of this treatment, the infant's nervous system was damaged and her physical development dwarfed for life. After bringing suit against both author and publisher, this mother received a settlement of $150,000—small compensation for the irreparable harm that was innocently fostered by a parent's effort to keep her child "healthy."

Some years ago it was discovered that ointments containing a small amount of vitamin A were sometimes effective in treating, though not curing, teenage acne. In the zealous hope of completely eradicating the condition, many teens have been giving themselves daily doses of high-potency vitamin A pills containing as much as 200,000 to 300,000 International Units—fifty or more times as much as the RDA. Having continued this regimen for several months, many of these youngsters fell prey to the devastating combinations of symptoms presented in the chart on page 231. A jaundiced appearance is not unusual as body fat turns increasingly yellow. In adults, prolonged use of excessive amounts can lead to the same symptoms as vitamin A deficiency: night blindness and other forms of vision impairment.

Overdosing with vitamin D can be more serious, or even fatal. Individual tolerances vary widely, but in persons with lower tolerances too much vitamin D can release calcium and phosphorus from bony tissues and redeposit them in the walls of the blood vessels, as well as in the heart, kidneys, bronchial passages, and elsewhere. Such conditions are *not* reversible; they cannot be corrected by merely discontinuing all vitamin D supplements. For this reason, the FDA has placed certain restrictions on vitamin D fortification of foods and on the amount permitted in any single supplement dose. But there is nothing to stop the pill lover from downing them by the handful. And cod-liver oil, the beloved vitamin D source of yesteryear, has returned to the scene in a choice of plain, mint, or cherry.

Pregnancy creates a particular area of concern. Traditionally, vitamin/mineral supplements have been routinely prescribed for pregnant women. In reasonable amounts, such supplements provide an "insurance policy" for the growing fetus and are unlikely to cause any particular harm. The problems arise when the mother-to-be—or, alas, sometimes her doctor—decides that superdoses will produce a superkid. Unfortunately, what too often occurs is just the opposite. While excesses of fat-soluble vitamins like A and D harbor the most potential danger because they are not easily eliminated from the body, other vitamins can also present difficulties.

For example, there is the question of what is known as "rebound scurvy" among newborns. It is possible that if the infant's mother consumed megadoses of vitamin C during pregnancy, she might create in the unborn child a tolerance, and then a dependence, on these massive amounts. After birth, with vitamin C intake reduced to normal levels, the baby might present all the symptoms of scurvy; that is, vitamin C deficiency. Conceivably, excessive amounts of other nutrients could produce similar rebound results.

The complexity of nutrient interactions is not a matter for amateurs—or self-professed professionals—to tamper with. As a brief example, a deficiency of folic acid will cause anemia. However, even slightly excessive amounts taken during pernicious anemia *without a sufficient amount of vitamin B_{12}* can result in spinal cord degeneration.

There are countless such examples. However necessary a vitamin or any other substance may be for the maintenance of life and good health, too much of anything can throw the entire system out of balance and cause it to malfunction. The chart below lists only some of the symptoms that have been observed from prolonged consumption of excessive amounts of vitamins. How many other cause/effect relationships remain unknown is purely a matter of speculation.

Symptoms Observed in Hypervitaminosis

Vitamin A	Headaches; lack of appetite, frequent vomiting; lethargy; irritability; menstrual difficulties; drying, cracking, and thickening of the skin; severe itching; loss of hair; enlarged liver and spleen and, more rarely, severe liver damage; intracranial pressure due to increased fluid in the brain; bone and joint pains; bone fragility with frequent fractures; increased bleeding tendency; retarded growth in children; increased susceptibility to illness.
Vitamin B_3 (Niacin)	Severe flushing, itching, and other skin disorders; gout; liver damage; ulcers; blood-sugar disturbances.
Vitamin C	Diarrhea, especially in children; diuresis, possibly forming crystals in the urine and contributing to other kidney problems; damage to growing bones; rebound scurvy; adverse effects during pregnancy. May cause false positive urine tests for sugar in diabetics. Large doses can destroy substantial amounts of vitamin B_{12} in food, leading to a dangerous deficiency. (It does not prevent the common cold but in some cases appears to slightly reduce symptoms.)
Vitamin D	Nausea; weakness; loss of appetite; weight loss; constipation or diarrhea; vague aches and stiffness; calcification of tissues; abnormal bone growth in children; numbness and tingling of the bones and fingertips; high blood pressure; excessive urination; acidosis and kidney damage with possible kidney failure that can lead to death.
Vitamin E	Headaches; nausea; giddiness; general fatigue; muscle weakness; low blood sugar; blurred vision; chapped lips and inflammation of the mouth; gastrointestinal disturbances; increased bleeding tendency; degenerative changes; *reduced* sexual-organ function. (Results opposite of the last were obtained only in experiments conducted with laboratory rats.)

NATURAL VITAMINS

The case for "natural" vitamins is obscure at best. Extracted, desiccated, hydrolyzed, pressed into pills and placed into bottles does not sound very natural. But the point is moot. We have already discussed the fact that a synthetic vitamin is chemically identical to its counterpart found in nature. They function in precisely the same way, and they present the same problems of overdosing. Contrary to what you may occasionally hear, megadosing with natural vitamins is no "safer" than with the synthetics.

Furthermore, many of the natural vitamin preparations are little more than natural hoaxes. A supplement purporting to contain "vitamin C from natural rose hips," for instance, may in reality contain only a small percentage of vitamin C from that source, with the major portion as synthetic as in many other preparations. Analysis has occasionally revealed that little of a given nutrient was actually derived from its alleged natural source.

If you truly prefer natural vitamins, they are widely available in fruits, vegetables, breads, cereals, meats, and dairy products, and they cost far less than the so-called "natural preparation."

The Nonvitamins

The word "vitamin" is derived from *vita,* meaning life, and amine, a class of chemical substances originally thought to be components of all the vitamins. When this did not prove to be the case, the word was changed from the original vitamine to vitamin. Nonvitamins are not only nonessential, they may actually be harmful, either directly or indirectly.

Probably the most notorious of these nonvitamin frauds is Laetrile, which has masqueraded as "vitamin B_{17}." Widespread research revealing Laetrile to be a totally useless cancer "cure" should have laid it to rest finally and forever. But we cannot be so optimistic. There still remain, and perhaps always will, a few quacks eager to exchange worthless treatment for a desperate victim's dollars.

Almost equally as well known as Laetrile is pangamic acid, which travels under the guise of "vitamin B_{15}." Scientists aren't even sure exactly what chemical substance pangamic acid is, since combinations of a variety of substances, some of which are of questionable safety, have been found in containers labeled "B-15." But it is known that, like Laetrile, pangamic acid is not a vitamin; it is unnecessary in the diet and as a supplement is a waste of money, perhaps even potentially harmful.

Dr. Victor Herbert, clinical professor of medicine at the State University of New York Downstate Medical Center and director of the Hematology and Nutrition Laboratory at the Bronx Veterans Administration Medical Center and a nationally known expert on nutrition fraud, has investigated the B-15 problem extensively. He says that B-15 is a label, not a substance. Each seller tosses whatever chemicals he chooses into bottles labeled "B-15" or "pangamate." Not a single product has yet been found by the FDA to conform to the alleged chemical formula specified by B-15's creator.

Dr. Herbert also reports that the creator is a twice-convicted criminal of health fraud and is "doctor" by dint of an honorary doctorate in science from a small, now defunct Bible college in Oklahoma, which had no science department and no authority to award the degee.

The Food and Drug Administration considers the sale of B-15 or pangamic acid as a dietary supplement or drug illegal because there is no evidence that the substance is a vitamin, has therapeutic value, or is safe for human consumption. Nevertheless, when the product is available, it still sells well.

Why does B-15 sell so well? Dr. Herbert notes that B-15 has been promoted extensively through the use of "testimonials" from individuals who claim to have experienced its benefits. The FDA is powerless to prevent this kind of promotion, even though testimonials are worthless as evidence of safety or usefulness.

Dr. Herbert is also concerned about potentially toxic chemicals that have been found in some samples of "B-15." One such chemical may even be a cancer-causing agent.

Since many different ingredients have been found in containers labeled "B-15," the product is clearly inaccurately labeled. This *is* illegal. Investigators from the American Council on Science and Health followed up the mislabeling problem by writing to the promoters of B-15 and asking them to explain the inconsistency between what they said their product contained and what was really in it. Apparently, they struck a nerve.

In answer to the inquiry, investigators were told that ". . . since we do not officially recognize the [Council] as anything more than a group of individuals whose knee-jerk response originated with big business and big medicine's political manipulation, we have no intention of spending any more of our time or resources in processing your requests.

"We have real good answers to your obvious political questions, and we welcome an opportunity to air them in an open forum as opposed to the vagaries of personal correspondence. So when you are ready to meet with us out in the open and play out in the open as we have, we will be glad to answer your questions. Until such time, I suggest you check this information elsewhere."

The investigators, who thought they had "played out in the open" by identifying themselves in their letters as staffers of a nonprofit health organization, took the promoters' suggestion and checked elsewhere.

Specifically, they checked with the U.S. District Court for Northern Illinois. On October 28, 1980, Judge Stanley J. Roszkowski of this court condemned Aangamik-15 Calcium Pangamate tablets (a trade name for B-15) as adulterated and misbranded. In doing so, he upheld the FDA's seizure of six shipments of this product.

The judge based his decision on the language of the federal Food, Drug, and Cosmetic Act, which prohibits the mislabeling of food. Judge Roszkowski wrote, "It is uncontested that the Aangamik-15 tablets . . . are not a vitamin or a pro-vitamin." He added that there was no scientifically recognized vitamin B_{15} and that the tablets did not contain vitamin B_{15}. Further, the court found that the company which manufactured and distributed the tablets, Food Science Laboratories of South Burlington, Vermont, failed to list even the principal ingredients on the product label.

It appears that the "real good answers" the promoters claimed to have to the American Council investigators' questions about B-15 were not so good after all.

"Vitamin P" is rutin, a substance of no scientifically proved usefulness, and thus not a vitamin. Yet rutin is currently a highly touted dietary supplement. Carefully worded ads proclaim that it "is believed to be" an important component of the vitamin C complex, whatever that is, and that it "may be" the natural protection everybody is searching for.

"Vitamin T" is described in the *Dictionary of Health and Nutrition* as "an obscure vitamin whose composition is not known."

The same source also mentions "vitamin U," but the total information offered is the following: "A recently discovered factor in cabbage leaves and other green vegetables which has shown promising results in the treatment of ulcers." We can safely assume that dietary supplements are not required.

Nonvitamins or not, at least some of the above are peddled by the health-food hucksters as "necessary" for good health. And gullible consumers continue to buy them.

Minerals

Mineral supplements have been growing in popularity of late, possibly because of the relative novelty of many of them. While the majority of today's consumers probably grew up hearing at least vague references to the importance of iron and calcium, other minerals like magnesium, potassium, chromium, zinc, and selenium were generally awarded relatively little attention, if any at all. That is also a major reason the pill peddlers are able to get away with so much balderdash.

Minerals are not the complex structures that vitamins are; they are simple primary elements. Lacking carbon, they cannot by definition be called "organic." To refer to any of them as "natural" is equally absurd: They are always natural, since it is impossible to manufacture any basic element synthetically in the laboratory (unless you have a nuclear reactor in your lab). Likewise, the term "chelated mineral" is meaningless, (used to describe minerals that are claimed to carry undesirable substances out of the body) other than to produce one more method of jacking up prices.

About twenty or so mineral elements are known to be biologically necessary to human life, although the precise functions of some are still rather obscure.* Most of these are so widely available and required in such minuscule amounts that no RDA has ever been established. With the exceptions of iron and fluoride, mineral deficiencies are practically unheard of in the United States. And, as with vitamins, a mineral supplement can correct only a mineral deficiency. But scanning a few health-food ads would have us believe otherwise:

"Most diets are known to be zinc deficient. . . . Zinc serves as a vital element for maintaining the integrity of the skin, glands, enzymes, and other life functions."

Extra magnesium, we are told, is needed "to nourish the cells of the body."

Potassium "to help relax and normalize the system."

Manganese "to aid in building a stronger resistance."

One particularly flowery ad reads: "Out of the mysteries of the ocean comes . . . a natural and unadulterated extract from the green-lipped mussel" to "put the ocean's natural mineral balance to work for you."

---

* One health-food brochure refers to the presence of *sixty* different minerals in the human body, but it fails to identify them, and we are at a loss as to what all of them may be.

The subhead for a health food article on chromium reads: "Cleaner arteries and better handling of blood sugar may both be possible with this exciting mineral."

Selenium seems to be receiving the most attention of all. "Essential for the performance of vitally important physiological functions!" screams one ad. "Selenium is nature's great substance known to be important to your health," cries another. And, of course, most of them claim the product to be "certified natural."

A CLOSER LOOK

Calcium, phosphorus, magnesium. During the past few years a favorite source for calcium supplementation has been bone meal, a substance widely promoted by the health-food business and which also contains substantial amounts of phosphorus, magnesium, and lead. In 1977 the *Journal of the American Medical Association* reported the case history of a woman suffering from bone-meal-induced lead poisoning. An immediate random sampling of a number of bone-meal products from various health-food stores revealed that all were contaminated with lead in some degree. The reason is obvious: Most bone meal is processed in glue factories from horse bones. The bones of horses, and other animals, act as a reservoir for the deposit of excess lead; the older the horse, the greater the amount of lead. And only old horses go to glue factories.

Small amounts of lead are unavoidably introduced into the diet. Most is excreted in the urine; the rest gradually accumulates, usually in the bones. Lead has no known biological function, but in excessive amounts its toxic effects are well known. Unfortunately, particularly among adults, the symptoms of lead poisoning are often overlooked by physicians until the condition is far advanced. To overcome the stigma associated with old horses, bone meal today is usually advertised as originating from "100 percent imported beef" and "selected young healthy cattle." Whether such sources are always completely free from lead contamination is, however, questionable.

Those who preferred to skip the hazards of bone meal may have switched to dolomite, a mineral compound offering both calcium and magnesium "drawn from the heart of the earth." However, dolomite has also presented toxicity problems. In early 1981, two reports in the *New England Journal of Medicine* indicated that potentially toxic quantities of heavy metals could be found in some samples of dolomite.

The truth is that no one on a balanced diet requires supplements of calcium or magnesium. Even when calcium intake is borderline, or somewhat low, the metabolic system compensates by increasing its absorption efficiency—up to as much as double the percentage it would normally absorb from an optimally balanced diet.

As for magnesium, a deficiency is most unlikely because that mineral is found in *all* foods. The single exception is among children fed solely on milk, which is relatively low in magnesium. But anyone subsisting on only milk has a great many other problems to contend with. If you want to increase your magnesium intake, eat more whole grain products and potatoes, and don't waste your money on a magnesium dietary supplement.

Phosphorus, while present in bone meal, is not found in dolomite. But here again, deficiencies are virtually unknown because phosphorus is contained in so many foods. The mineral has had a somewhat colorful history, however. Early in the century, after it was discovered that the human brain contained a considerable amount of it, a college professor named Louis Agassiz extolled the virtues of eating fish, since its high phosphorus content would allegedly make one think better. In *The New Nuts Among the Berries,* Ronald Deutsch related a follow-up anecdote: In the magazine *Galaxy,* Mark Twain was once queried on the subject by a "young author." Twain's answer: "Yes, Agassiz does recommend authors to eat fish. . . . But I cannot help you to a decision about the amount you need to eat—at least, with certainty. If the specimen composition you sent is about your fair, usual average, I should judge that perhaps a couple of whales would be all you would want for the present."

Of course, Mark Twain was not a nutritionist, either. But he undoubtedly possessed as much knowledge, and more intelligence, than most of the self-styled "specialists"—then or now.

Iron. The greatest problem surrounding iron intake is that the body is able to absorb and utilize only about 10 percent of what is consumed. Among women of childbearing age, iron deficiency occurs rather frequently. Extra care should be taken to include iron-rich foods regularly in the diet, but this does not mean you need a daily dose of either desiccated liver or liver juice. Iron supplements should be taken only on the advice of a physician and based on laboratory tests. It is wise not to exceed the recommended dosage. Disorders can result from too much iron just as well as from too little. There are cases on record where individuals have been fatally poisoned by excessive amounts of iron supplements. People who keep multivitamin/mineral tablets in the house should be aware of this. Many such preparations contain iron, especially the products that are advertised for women. Because of their iron content, these tablets are potentially poisonous for small children and should be kept out of reach, like all medicines.

Sodium and potassium. Statistics show that most Americans consume from ten to thirty times more sodium than they need, most of it in the form of sodium chloride (table salt). Potassium is widely available in foods and has never presented a deficiency problem for normal Americans. Unfortunately, the converse is not true. According to a report in *Medical World News,* Adelle Davis' book *Let's Have Healthy Children* led to still another tragedy when a Florida couple, following her recommendation, gave their child large doses of potassium as treatment for colic. After being given 2,500 mg of potassium chloride on one day and 500 mg the next, the infant suffered cardiac arrest and died. The attending physician, who was also then director of Pediatric Intensive Care at Jackson Memorial Hospital in Miami, cited potassium overdose as the probable cause of death and noted that the child "got at least four or five times the safe amount of potassium."

One of the rare circumstances in which potassium supplements are necessary is for astronauts during space travel. The absence of gravity tends to cause potassium to "leak" out of the cells and be excreted in the urine, creating a temporary deficiency. People who take certain medications, such as some diuretics used in the treatment of high blood pressure, may also need potassium supplements; that is, if foods rich in potassium, such as bananas, cannot supply adequate potassium. In this case, the supplements would be prescribed by the physician. But claims that "everyone could benefit" from potassium supplementation or that potassium will "relieve fatigue" are nonsense.

Iodide and fluoride. Iodide in plants, like most other minerals, depends on the soil content of the minerals. In certain parts of the United States, most notably in the Great Lakes region, iodide *is* deficient in the soil, and thus *it tends to be* deficient in the diet. In earlier times, when most food was locally grown, iodide-deficient food frequently resulted in goiter. Because of this deficit, iodized salt came into production in 1924, and goiter caused by iodide deficiency among Americans became a thing of the past. For whatever peculiar reason, during recent years iodide in salt has been dismissed as an "artificial additive," and much of the salt now available in stores is no longer iodized. Many institutions, such as schools and hospitals, have unfortunately discontinued use of iodized salt in their kitchens. Many health-food proponents maintain satisfactory levels of iodide by squandering money on relatively expensive sea salt and kelp with their "naturally occurring" iodide. The issue is not only potentially health-damaging (from too much iodide), it is downright silly. There is no such thing as "synthetic iodide." And iodide overdosing, easily possible with kelp tablets, is as harmful as receiving too little iodide.

A relative of iodide, fluoride is a mineral necessary for the protection of both teeth and bones. Our diets are low in fluoride, and hence, as we have mentioned earlier, fluorides added to the community water supply have resulted in a remarkable reduction in tooth decay. Yet the antiadditive people remain obstinate. One writer accused: "The stuff they put in your drinking water is also used to kill lice on chickens." The reasoning behind this statement is analogous to using an entire box of salt for seasoning a small hamburger, and it makes just about as much sense.

The sad and frustrating part of all this is that many of the same people who decry the use of iodide and fluoride as "artificial additives" are the same ones who advocate megadoses of other nutrients that not only are unnecessary but may actually be harmful. The paradox is unfathomable.

Selenium. Despite its featured prominence in so many health-food ads, this trace mineral is not a nutrient without which your body is barely surviving. A selenium/vitamin E compound has been touted as a cure for cancer, heart disease, and myriad other ills under the theory that it acts as a "scavenger" to protect the nucleic acids in body cells. Preposterous.

Selenium, except in the most minute amounts, is deadly. According to Dr. Theodore P. Labuza in *Food and Your Well-Being* (1977), deficiency diseases of either selenium or such other trace minerals as cadmium, nickel, tin, vanadium, and silicon "have never been found even experimentally." You can safely skip the selenium supplements.

Other trace minerals. Copper is another essential mineral that is extremely toxic in more than a minuscule amount and for which a true deficiency is almost unknown in our society. However, this small amount is necessary for the synthesis of hemoglobin.

Cobalt is a part of the vitamin B_{12} molecule and hence an essential mineral nutrient.

We have read much about zinc deficiency recently, and while some people think it may exist in our country, it is certainly not very common.

Chromium deficiency has been artificially produced in rats, but the likelihood of this occurring in humans—even on a diet that is not especially well balanced—is extremely remote. The amounts required by the body are so small, it is difficult to avoid consuming sufficient quantities. The same can be said for manganese and molybelenium.

More Wonder Foods

It is not only vitamin/mineral preparations that the health-foodists attempt to push on the public. There are any number of superfoods that are advocated as well, sometimes because they happen to be especially rich in one or another specific nutrient, although that is not a prerequisite. Palatability doesn't count.

To be fair, most health-food stores also offer an assortment of products that do sound tempting, such items as almond butter, rye flour, artichoke macaroni, for example, and unusual varieties of juices, jellies, and ice cream that are rarely available elsewhere and are certainly to be enjoyed if you like them and want to pay the prices. But there are other creations that make our stomachs quiver when we read the contents. Laxatives and diuretics, for example, that contain such ingredients as "ox bile" and "desiccated stomach substances" do not sound very appealing. Even so-called "natural" products often contain substances most skeptics would never be caught eating in processed foods.

Most of the "wonder foods" we will mention here, along with some of their outlandish claims, are old standbys. Since we are attempting to confine this book to one volume, we will not attempt to refute in detail all the allegations; we simply wish to point out the kind of nonsense to avoid, since few of the claims have any scientific basis or merit. We don't necessarily mean to imply you should avoid the products entirely, but you should be wary of fallacious pronouncements.

Alfalfa, the health quacks would have us believe, is truly a wonder food: "Contains every essential amino acid" ... "Antitoxin

properties unsurpassed" ... "Increases resistance to disease" ...
"Helps arthritis and other 'itises' " ... "Prevents exhaustion."
One writer offered the suggestion that as a food it might be better
with the fiber removed because it tended to "upset some people's
digestion." Little wonder, since at our present stage of evolution
the human stomach is ill equipped to handle such coarse roughage. While alfalfa is actually a good source of vitamins A and K,
there are more pleasant ways of obtaining these nutrients.

Kelp includes several types of ocean seaweed rich in iodide and
purported to "help bones heal faster." Some health foodists attribute fanciful properties to the weeds, insisting that any food
from the sea must contain "every essential factor necessary for
life." Not only is that faulty reasoning in itself, but scientists
know that many clams, mussels, and certain species of fish contain a naturally occurring enzyme that destroys thiamine. Further, at least a few partakers of kelp tablets have suffered arsenic
poisoning from overindulging. Presumably there is small likelihood that one would actually eat too much of the real thing. (If
you wish to bypass both weed and pills, there is kelp incense—
but no known claim for its contribution to human nutrition.)

Blackstrap molasses dates at least as far back as the Renaissance,
although it was then known as treacle or theriaca. In the sixteenth century it was touted as a cure for plague, but the myths
compounded themselves, and by the eighteenth century it was
reputed to be good for all ailments. It is worth noting that much
of its popularity at that time may have been due to the fact that it
was usually taken with wine. Blackstrap's overblown reputation
has persisted to the point where it is now held in high esteem
among health faddists as a source of minerals, particularly iron,
and calcium and B vitamins, and is credited with restoring hair
color, preventing anemia, and even stopping falling hair. As a
source of B vitamins, blackstrap is not very impressive; 42.5 tablespoons would be needed to fulfill the RDA for riboflavin, 50
tablespoons for niacin, and 75 tablespoons—or over 3,200
calories—for thiamine.

Fructose ads tell us this sugar is "twice as sweet as table sugar so you will lose weight." Evidently, the reasoning here is that only half as much is required to achieve the level of sweetness provided by ordinary table sugar or sucrose. But this is true only in cold foods. In your coffee, for instance, fructose and sucrose have equal sweetening power. Given the limited conditions under which such a substitution is possible, this seems like an exceedingly slow method of weight reduction. Undaunted, however, manufacturers now have fructose candies available in strawberry, banana, and spearmint flavors. (See chapter 7 for further discussion of fructose.)

Honey—natural, unrefined, unclarified, unheated—is still promoted as "nature's own sweetener." Rarely does one encounter any mention of the possible dangers from wild honey made by bees feeding on poisonous plants. (Honey has been discussed in greater detail in chapter 7.)

Apple-cider vinegar, alone or combined with honey, will probably never go out of style. Aside from preventing or curing almost any condition that might ail you, this vinegar is alleged necessary to keep the body from becoming too alkaline, because a "constant state of alkalinity contributes to cancer." It is also said to "keep the blood thin," thus improving circulation and at the same time lessening the "inclination to bleed." (If there appears to be a contradiction there, don't let it trouble you. Food faddists don't.) Further, apple-cider vinegar supposedly has the ability to control intestinal flora and render disease bacteria ineffective. How the substance is able to distinguish between the bad guys and the good guys of the digestive system is unknown.

Milk products. Other professed improvers of digestion are the various cultured milk products, the best known of which are *yogurt* and *acidophilus* dairy products (usually milk and cottage cheese). Acidophilus is also sold in tablet form. As with apple-cider vinegar, these cultures theoretically act to "stabilize the intestinal flora" and "eliminate putrefaction," because the disturb-ing bacteria can't survive in the presence of lactic acid. *Whey* tablets are likewise alleged to "help absorption of vitamins and minerals" and "sweeten the intestinal tract." *Kefir* is usually taken in liquid form but as a solid has the consistency of yogurt and is said to be "hygienic" for the digestive system. Additionally, since 1907, yogurt has been advocated for lengthening the life span, and Adelle Davis and company have often declared yogurt responsible for the supposedly unusual good health of the Bulgarians.

Of course, cultured dairy product such as yogurt, acidophilus milk, and kefir are perfectly good foods. They provide the nutrients of milk, and many people like their special tastes and textures. But they have no magical medical properties.

During the past decade, *bran* has been credited with a variety of health-giving properties. In moderation it helps to prevent constipation; in excess it can contribute to a variety of problems, perhaps the most important of which is its ability to bind with iron and render it unavailable for use. Even some of the health faddists are aware of this iron-building quality, so the latest ploy is to recommend enzyme supplements to help absorption of iron or to substitute sprouts (which have less fiber than bran), although the reasoning is a bit fuzzy.

Sprouts may be those of mung beans, soybeans, alfalfa seeds, or other plants. The claim here is that when the seeds sprout, their vitamin content increases by as much as 1,000 percent. That is a little exaggerated, even though the nutrient content of sprouts is a little higher than that of the plant from which the sprout is grown.

Wheat germ, granola, and other "health" cereals have been around for a long time. Many of them are quite tasty, but check the labels before buying—several are more "natural" than they are nutritious and they are all hefty in calories, which is worth remembering if you're watching your weight.

Sunflower seeds are purported to be "invaluable for victims of hypoglycemia because they raise the blood sugar naturally through the protein content." Almost anyone can perceive that this contention is irrational. (A few generations ago, sunflower seeds and pumpkin seeds were used to "cure" tapeworm. With nothing else to eat, the worms were thought to soon starve to death.)

Raw gelatin is often promoted as an energy booster used by Lucille Ball and other stars. It *is* pure protein, but so lacking in some essential amino acids that almost any other food has better-quality protein. As an energy source it is no more useful than ordinary table sugar, and less efficient.

Protein supplements, in the form of tablets, powders, or liquids, seem to be particularly recommended for athletes these days, although the propaganda would have us believe that everyone can benefit from them. In reality, national surveys have revealed that even at poverty levels, Americans are getting 60 to 100 percent more protein than the National Research Council finds adequate. Other studies indicate that the average citizen receives three to five times as much as needed. After intensive investigation, the Federal Trade Commission has stated: "Protein deficiency is probably the least common of all major nutrient deficiencies in the U.S." Protein is readily available in foods—for athletes and nonathletes—yet many are paying up to twenty dollars per day and more for this and other health-food supplements. Physical exercise does not increase one's need for protein, only for calories and water.

Bee pollen is another favorite substance for the fortification of athletes. One ad cites its bee-pollen and wheat-germ combination as a "perfect marriage of nature." A company in Arizona selling bee pollen claims that President Reagan takes it daily, but we have inquired about that and obtained a negative answer.

246

Desiccated liver. Athletes are also the special target for the sale of *desiccated* (that is, dried) *liver,* but its wonders are presumably beneficial to every man, woman, and child. The theory here is that the liver acts as a depot for the storage of all vitamins and minerals and thus is a "powerhouse of nutrients." It is said not only to provide great stamina but to accomplish other wonders, such as recoloring prematurely gray hair. Liver juice is frequently recommended for diabetics, but the connection is unclear.

Lecithin has been a hot item for many years, an apparent panacea for both health and beauty. It is highly touted as a "specific antidote for cholesterol." Depending on which health-food sources you read, you will be told that lecithin "dissolves cholesterol" or keeps it in a "state of emulsion." The processes are not the same, but neither is true; nor is the further claim that the substance "dissolves the plaques of atherosclerosis." The fact is that lecithin is produced in the body in sufficient amounts and that supplementation is useless.

Brewer's yeast is heralded as a "superior natural additive," an all-time classic for you, your children, and your pets. As we have mentioned, it is an excellent source of B vitamins and protein, but there is nothing magical about it.

Papaya extract and its alleged mystical enzyme, *papain,* is another of the newer cure-alls. Among other things it is said to aid in the digestion of protein and alleviate other digestive problems, to cure pyorrhea, and promote weight reduction. We have already noted that enzymes ingested by mouth are quickly destroyed by stomach acids. About the only special thing that papaya extract can really do is to tenderize meat—outside of the digestive tract, of course. But we doubt that health-food enthusiasts would approve of such an "unnatural" culinary practice.

Food Sources of Nutrients in Relation to United States Recommended Dietary Allowances*

	Sources†			
Nutrient	Excellent (75% U.S. RDA)	Good (50% U.S. RDA)	Significant (25% U.S. RDA)	Fair (10% U.S. RDA)
Ascorbic acid	Orange Strawberries Cauliflower Broccoli Br. sprouts Green pepper Tomato Grapefruit Honeydew melon Mustard greens	Cabbage Spinach Tangerine Asparagus	Banana Blueberries Lima beans Raspberries Green peas Radishes Sauerkraut	Apple Peach Corn
Vitamin A	Liver Carrot Pumpkin Sweet potatoes Spinach Winter squash Turnip greens Mustard greens Beet greens	Apricots Watermelon Broccoli	Honeydew melon Peaches Prunes Tomato Nectarines	Asparagus Green beans Br. sprouts Cheddar cheese Green peas Tomato juice
Thiamine	Pork	Dried peas Macaroni	Green peas Ham Peanuts	Orange Watermelon Dried beans Noodles Spaghetti Lamb liver Rice Cashew nuts

248

Riboflavin	Liver	Macaroni, Cottage cheese, Buttermilk, Milk, Yogurt		Avocado, Tangerine, Prunes, Asparagus, Broccoli, Mushrooms, Ice cream, Beef, Salmon, Turkey
Vitamin B_6	Soybeans, Beef liver, Tuna	Lima beans, Pork, Beef, Veal, Halibut, Salmon, Chicken, Bananas, Avocado		Cauliflower, Green pepper, Potatoes, Spinach, Raisins, Perch
Vitamin B_{12}	Beef liver, Clams, Salmon, Trappist cheese, Lamb, Eggs	Veal, Cheese, Scallops, Swordfish		
Magnesium	Molasses, Peanuts	Spinach, Lima beans, Green peas	Beet greens	Raisins, Sweet potatoes, Br. sprouts, Cod

Food Sources of Nutrients in Relation to United States Recommended Dietary Allowances*

	Sources†			
Nutrient	Excellent (75% U.S. RDA)	Good (50% U.S. RDA)	Significant (25% U.S. RDA)	Fair (10% U.S. RDA)
Iron	Calves' and pork liver Clams	Beef liver	Asparagus Ham Veal Beef Chicken Macaroni Prunes Raisins Spinach	Banana Beans Br. sprouts Cod Green peas Noodles Rice Cashew nuts Peanuts
Calcium			Turnip greens Swiss cheese Buttermilk Milk Yogurt Salmon	Prunes Broccoli Beet greens Cottage cheese Ice cream Haddock Scallops

* From Helen A. Guthrie, *Introductory Nutrition*, 4th edition, (St. Louis: The C.V. Mosby Company, 1979).
† Based on average serving size as follows:
Meat—3 oz, edible portion
Fruit—3 to 4 oz
Vegetables—3 to 4 oz
Cereals—1 oz
Milk—8 oz

Ginseng root has appeared as a favorite instrument of the occult for centuries. The name derives from two Chinese characters meaning "man-plant," since the root often appears to have arms and legs, thus assuming the vague shape of a rather deformed-looking man. Some ads "guarantee" a "joyful temper, plenty of pure red blood, and relief for your irritable bladder," and cite testimonials from users who claim "increased energy and vigor." Others make no medical claims at all, stating only that it is not harmful. Be wary of literature promising that ginseng will cure heart disease, stroke, diabetes, digestive problems, stress, fatigue, or nervous disorders. There is no scientific evidence that it has any effect on such conditions, or that it is an aphrodisiac, as many rumors claim.

Herbal teas. The use of *herbal teas* in all varieties dates back to ancient Chinese and Greek cultures. Dozens of varieties are available today, either at health-food stores or by direct mail. Carefully worded literature suggests which combination of herbs to use for every imaginable ailment but makes no actual promises of cure. As mentioned in chapter 5, many of these herbs represent potential drug-abuse problems or may be harmful in other ways. They should be approached with extreme caution, if at all. Think of herbs the way you think of wild mushrooms. An expert can select the safe ones, but most of us can't.

The list goes on. We have included here most of the major products, but health-food manufacturers are unlikely ever to run out of ways to separate the gullible from their money.

Beauty Treatments and the Fountain of Youth

Youth and beauty are highly valued commodities, and how well the health-food merchants know that. Not content merely to stuff our stomachs with superfoods, they have devised all manner of cosmetic aids: yogurt face cream and body powder, turtle-oil wrinkle remover, mint-julep face mask, placenta shampoo,

Foods Which Are Important Sources of Vitamins and Minerals*

Nutrient	Food†	
	Excellent source (over 50% U.S. RDA)	*Good source* (25% to 50% U.S. RDA)
Vitamin A	Liver, calf Liver, chicken Carrots Pumpkin Spinach Sweet potato Cantaloupe Mixed vegetables Winter squash Broccoli Apricots Pepper, red Plums, canned	Tomatoes, cooked Watermelon
Vitamin C	Citrus fruits or juices Broccoli Pepper, red or green Brussels sprouts Cantaloupe Strawberries Cauliflower Tomatoes or juice Cabbage Spinach, cooked Asparagus Honeydew melon	Liver, calf Lima beans Potato, baked Blackberries Raspberries Watermelon
Thiamine	Pork loin Pork loin chop	Pork, cured or fresh Ham Foods made with enriched flour Spareribs Soybeans Cereal, ready-to-eat (check label) Peas
Riboflavin	Liver, calf Liver, chicken	Cheese, cottage Milk Custard Yogurt Ice milk Pudding Welsh rarebit Foods made with enriched flour Cereals, ready-to-eat (check labels)

Niacin	Peanuts (1 cup)	Turkey
	Liver	Fish
	Chicken	Veal
	Tuna	Pork
		Beef
		Lamb
		Sardines
		Foods made with enriched flour
Calcium		Milk
		Custard
		Yogurt
		Pudding
		Cheese
		Sardines
		Macaroni and cheese
Iron	Liver	Meats
	Farina, enriched, cooked	Beans
	Prunes	Lentils
		Soybeans
		Dates
		Raisins
		Apricots, dried
		Peaches, dried

* Adapted from Fredrick J. Stare, M.D., and Margaret McWilliams, Ph.D., *Living Nutrition*, 3rd edition, (New York: John Wiley and Sons, 1980).
† Based on average servings as follows:
Meat—3 oz. edible portion
Vegetable—1 cup
Fruit—3 to 4 oz.
Cereal—1 oz.
Legumes or Pasta—1 cup cooked
Milk—1 cup

"therapeutic" bath oil, papaya and oatmeal soaps, royal bee jelly, spearmint-leaf body scrub, kelp cleansers, ginseng face cream, dolomite toothpaste, and a mud pack described as "a natural earth facial" that retails at three dollars for a six-ounce jar.

Deodorants are available in scents ranging from mint to citrus. Hair restorers are rampant, one of which lists "57 specific ingredients," chockful of vitamins and minerals. Vitamin E can be found in every sort of medium, from creams, lotions, and ointments to soaps, shampoos, and face powders. Then there is Dr. Kilmer's Swamp Root, an herbal diuretic in a 10 percent alcohol base.

Of course, the hucksters are perfectly willing to sell us an array

FOOD AND NUTRITION BOARD, NATIONAL ACADEMY OF SCIENCES-NATIONAL RESEARCH COUNCIL RECOMMENDED DAILY DIETARY ALLOWANCES, Revised 1980

Designed for the maintenance of good nutrition of practically all healthy people in the U.S.A.

	Age (years)	Weight (kg)	Weight (lb)	Height (cm)	Height (in)	Protein (g)	Fat-Soluble Vitamins Vitamin A (µg RE)[b]	Vitamin D (µg)[c]	Vitamin E (mg α-TE)[d]	Water-Soluble Vitamins Vitamin C (mg)	Thiamine (mg)	Riboflavin (mg)	Niacin (mg NE)[e]	Vitamin B-6 (mg)	Folacin[f] (µg)	Vitamin B-12 (µg)	Minerals Calcium (mg)	Phosphorus (mg)	Magnesium (mg)	Iron (mg)	Zinc (mg)	Iodine (µg)
Infants	0.0-0.5	6	13	60	24	kg × 2.2	420	10	3	35	0.3	0.4	6	0.3	30	0.5[g]	360	240	50	10	3	40
	0.5-1.0	9	20	71	28	kg × 2.0	400	10	4	35	0.5	0.6	8	0.6	45	1.5	540	360	70	15	5	50
Children	1-3	13	29	90	35	23	400	10	5	45	0.7	0.8	9	0.9	100	2.0	800	800	150	15	10	70
	4-6	20	44	112	44	30	500	10	6	45	0.9	1.0	11	1.3	200	2.5	800	800	200	10	10	90
	7-10	28	62	132	52	34	700	10	7	45	1.2	1.4	16	1.6	300	3.0	800	800	250	10	10	120
Males	11-14	45	99	157	62	45	1000	10	8	50	1.4	1.6	18	1.8	400	3.0	1200	1200	350	18	15	150
	15-18	66	145	176	69	56	1000	10	10	60	1.4	1.7	18	2.0	400	3.0	1200	1200	400	18	15	150
	19-22	70	154	177	70	56	1000	7.5	10	60	1.5	1.7	19	2.2	400	3.0	800	800	350	10	15	150
	23-50	70	154	178	70	56	1000	5	10	60	1.4	1.6	18	2.2	400	3.0	800	800	350	10	15	150
	51+	70	154	178	70	56	1000	5	10	60	1.2	1.4	16	2.2	400	3.0	800	800	350	10	15	150
Females	11-14	46	101	157	62	46	800	10	8	50	1.1	1.3	15	1.8	400	3.0	1200	1200	300	18	15	150
	15-18	55	120	163	64	46	800	10	8	60	1.1	1.3	14	2.0	400	3.0	1200	1200	300	18	15	150
	19-22	55	120	163	64	44	800	7.5	8	60	1.1	1.3	14	2.0	400	3.0	800	800	300	18	15	150
	23-50	55	120	163	64	44	800	5	8	60	1.0	1.2	13	2.0	400	3.0	800	800	300	18	15	150
	51+	55	120	163	64	44	800	5	8	60	1.0	1.2	13	2.0	400	3.0	800	800	300	10	15	150
Pregnant						+30	+200	+5	+2	+20	+0.4	+0.3	+2	+0.6	+400	+1.0	+400	+400	+150	h	+5	+25
Lactating						+20	+400	+5	+3	+40	+0.5	+0.5	+5	+0.5	+100	+1.0	+400	+400	+150	h	+10	+50

a The allowances are intended to provide for individual variations among most normal persons as they live in the United States under usual environmental stresses. Diets should be based on a variety of common foods in order to provide other nutrients for which human requirements have been less well defined.

b Retinol equivalents. 1 retinol equivalent = 1 µg retinol or 6 µg β carotene. See text for calculation of vitamin A activity of diets as retinol equivalents.

c As cholecalciferol. 10 µg cholecalciferol = 400 IU of vitamin D.

d α-tocopherol equivalents. 1 mg d-α tocopherol = 1 α-TE.

e 1 NE (niacin equivalent) is equal to 1 mg of niacin or 60 mg of dietary tryptophan.

f The folacin allowances refer to dietary sources as determined by *Lactobacillus casei* assay after treatment with enzymes (conjugases) to make polyglutamyl forms of the vitamin available to the test organism.

g The recommended dietary allowance for vitamin B$_{12}$ in infants is based on average concentration of the vitamin in human milk. The allowances after weaning are based on energy intake (as recommended by the American Academy of Pediatrics) and consideration of other factors, such as intestinal absorption.

h The increased requirement during pregnancy cannot be met by the iron content of habitual American diets nor by the existing iron stores of many women: therefore the use of 30–60 mg of supplemental iron is recommended. Iron needs during lactation are not substantially different from those of nonpregnant women, but continued supplementation of mother for 2–3 months after parturition is advisable in order to replenish stores, depleted by the pregnancy.

of supplements as well, and there are a number of unknowledgeable "beauty" writers helping to spread the propaganda. Thus, we read that extra vitamin A promotes nail growth, riboflavin protects against baldness, niacin eliminates bad breath, vitamin B deficiency causes dandruff, pantothenic acid prevents aging, potassium helps maintain a healthy skin, ad infinitum.

Good health—outside and inside—is promoted by a healthful, balanced diet. Dietary supplements and expensive "health" cosmetic preparations will have little effect on the way you look. As for the Fountain of Youth, if it is ever discovered, we hope to be first in line for a dip.

Recommendations

A maxim of pharmacology states that anything causing bodily changes for good can also do the opposite. This elementary principle can be applied as accurately to vitamins, minerals, and other nutrients as it is to medicinal drugs.

There is always a point of maximum effectiveness; beyond that point lies the risk of toxic effects. Further danger exists in the fact that a large dose of one nutrient sometimes blocks the body's ability to use another. Those who succumb to the vitamin-quack sales talk should realize they are taking part in a large, uncontrolled experiment.

People are often distressed to learn that the concept of a miracle potion simply doesn't stand up; they prefer to cling to their fantasies, rather than bother themselves about balanced diets and other simple and relatively inexpensive aspects of healthful living. Our contention that, in the absence of deficiency disease, almost everyone can obtain all necessary nutrients from regular, varied selections from the Basic Four Food Groups is not very spectacular. Certainly, it will not create world-shaking headlines. But it is based on sound scientific facts.

In nutrient intake, the objective is, like salt for the stew, not too little, not too much.

CHAPTER 9

You Are What You Eat: Nutrition and Behavior

Are You What You Eat?

"TELL ME WHAT YOU EAT, AND I WILL TELL you what you are." This statement was first attributed to Anthelme Brillat-Savarin, a French lawyer and politician, some 150 years ago.

In a sense, yes, you are what you eat. A well-balanced diet contributes a great deal to good health, and good health certainly influences how you feel and react toward others. But except for certain sensitivities to some foods,* the idea that a specific food or nutrient has any direct effect on personality or behavior is absurd. The theory makes about as much sense as saying scrambled eggs will make you cackle when you laugh, or that eating prunes will give you wrinkles.

* It is to be understood that this exception holds throughout this chapter. A few persons do have a sensitivity or intolerance for some foods that may indirectly influence behavior. But such sensitivity should be medically determined by testing and is quite uncommon.

256

Primitive man believed he took on the attributes of mals he ate, thus preferring to partake of the brave l' than the timid deer. While such archaic thinking is *1* typical in our atomic age, nevertheless, there is no related nonsense.

Immorality at the Dinner Table

An 1861 cookbook, *Christianity in the Kitchen,* by Mrs. Horace Mann, opened with the enticing sentence, "There's death in the pot." Farther along, Mrs. Mann wrote: "There is no more prolific cause of bad morals than abuses of diet."

More than a century later, this same line of thought is still being served up as though it were brand new. In *Psychodietetics,* a book by dentists Emanuel Cheraskin and W. M. Ringsdorf, Jr., and Arline Brecher, the authors proclaim, "Deteriorating eating habits share a major responsibility in the rise of violence in our population today." Adelle Davis carried this notion even further by stating: "Alcoholism, crime, insanity, suicide, divorce, drug addiction, and even impotency are often merely the results of bad eating."

"Good" eating to the health faddists generally seems to mean only organically grown foods, plus a few bottles of vitamins and other pepper-uppers from the health-food store; to be avoided at all costs are processed foods and almost everything white, like bread and sugar. Even milk has been accused of causing autism in children. In *Killer Salt,* Marietta Whittlesey writes that salt causes depression. (Excessive use of salt can be harmful in other ways, but there is no evidence that it affects the psyche.)

There are still many individuals who agree with Sylvester Graham's old contention that meat increases man's animal appetites and makes him violent—a theory that tends to be punched out by the fact that Hitler and Mussolini were both vegetarians.

What all of this boils down to is a giant cop-out. That line of reasoning would give license to anyone to do anything. Placing the blame on food is the same as saying one isn't responsible for his or her own actions—a marvelous built-in excuse for unhitching all inner controls.

The prospect is frightening—and becomes more so as the diet-behavior concept is increasingly expanded by the health gurus, including a few doctors. Now lawyers, too, are hopping on the bandwagon as they defend clients by claiming that their criminal behavior was caused by hypoglycemia or some dietary deficiency.

Hyperkinesis and Dr. Ben Feingold

Between 5 and 10 percent of all school-age children in the United States have been labeled "hyperactive," or, in medical terminology, "hyperkinetic." The hyperactive child is of normal intelligence but has great difficulty in sitting still or concentrating. He or she disrupts the family and creates havoc in the classroom.

Many theories on the cause of hyperkinesis have been presented, but none has been proven, and no fully effective treatment exists. As a result, the condition is a terribly frustrating problem for its young victims, parents, and teachers.

One of the first major theories of modern times linking diet and behavior was born in 1973 when the late Dr. Ben Feingold, a California pediatric allergist, proposed that salicylates (naturally occurring compounds present in many fruits, some vegetables, and a number of other foods), together with artificial colors and flavors, were among the causes of hyperkinesis. He suggested a diet free of these substances as treatment and prevention of the condition. In essence, that meant the elimination of not only a great many vegetables and fruits, but all manufactured baked goods, luncheon meats, ice cream, powdered puddings, candies, soft drinks, tea, coffee, colored margarine, butter, and most commercially produced condiments. In addition, the theory demanded exclusion of many nonfood items such as toothpaste, mouthwash, cough drops, and some over-the counter and prescription drugs.

Dr. Feingold's theory on the cause and treatment of hyperkinesis gradually evolved and changed. His hypothesis regarding the relationship with diet began with his interpretation of research on aspirin intolerance in the early 1970s. Feingold pointed out that the chemical structure of salicylates, which occur naturally in many foods, is the same as that of aspirin. He proposed that hyperkinesis was a symptom of salicylate intolerance for food in genetically predisposed individuals, since the reaction is biochemically similar to aspirin hypersensitivity.

Because many aspirin-intolerant individuals also demonstrate a hypersensitivity to tartrazine (Yellow Dye #5),* Feingold further suggested that this additive was likewise related to hyperactivity. Noting that the chemical structure of several artificial flavors contains a component similar to that of the salicylates, he theorized that these additives, too, were involved.

Based on these observations and hypotheses, Dr. Feingold developed his theory on the treatment and prevention of hyperkinesis through diet and presented his ideas in a popular book, not, as is the usual custom, in a recognized medical or scientific journal. Forbidden foods included all those high in salicylates and all those containing artificial (synthetic) colors and/or flavors.

In more recent publications (again not in the medical literature), Dr. Feingold revised his recommendations. He came to believe that after four to six weeks the salicylate-containing foods can be returned to the diet of the hyperactive child if no adverse reactions occur. This change marks an important shift in the theory. Now the major emphasis is on the artificial additives, and the role of salicylates has been minimized. This change is very clear in Feingold's last publication on the subject, a cookbook. In it, BHA and BHT, two antioxidant additives that are commonly used in prepared foods in the United States, have been added to the list of chemicals Feingold believed related to

---

* Aspirin is one form of salicylate.

259

hyperactivity. He thus recommended that they, too, be eliminated from the diet, even though they have no chemical similarity to salicylates.

Dr. Feingold's recommendations have been adopted by the parents of many hyperactive children, with some reporting noticeable improvement in their child's behavior when the diet was carefully followed. Based on clinical observation and testimonials—not controlled scientific study—Feingold himself reported that nearly 48 to 50 percent of those who adhere strictly to his diet recommendations show a marked reduction in hyperactive behavior, and, of those who respond, two-thirds do so dramatically.

Eating in restaurants and school cafeterias is practically impossible on the Feingold diet. Convenience foods are generally restricted because they contain artificial colors and flavors. Homemade foods, prepared from "scratch," therefore become necessary for all family meals. Feingold strongly recommended including the hyperactive child in the food preparation and encouraged the entire family to participate in the diet program. Supposedly, this prevents the child from feeling "different," reduces temptation, and provides the positive motivation of "team" involvement. What it also does, of course, is to focus considerable attention on the child. Many physicians and scientists knowledgeable in this area believe that this extra attention is in itself responsible for improved behavior.

In any case, rigorous scientific tests of the Feingold hypothesis simply do not support his claims. Scientists who looked closely at Dr. Feingold's theory realized that some parts of it simply didn't make good scientific sense. The reason for excluding artificial food flavorings from the diet was unclear, because the chemical components of artificial flavors are usually identical to those found naturally in food. Since the human body doesn't distinguish between natural and synthetic substances that are chemically identical, it wouldn't be reasonable for a child to be sensitive to artificial vanilla flavor, for instance, and not to natural vanilla flavor. Also, different artificial flavors are made of many different chemicals, most of which are unrelated to each other. There is little reason to expect that this wide variety of substances could *all* cause the same reaction—hyperactive behavior.

The scientists also had questions about the salicylate part of the hypothesis. Dr. Feingold had specified a list of fruits and vegetables prohibited on the special diet because they contained salicylates. However, when food scientists measured the amount of salicylate in these foods, they found that some of the foods prohibited on the diet contained only very small amounts of salicylates, while some foods that were allowed contained large amounts.

For these reasons, tests of the Feingold hypothesis focused on food colors and on the diet as a whole. Salicylates and flavors were given less emphasis.

Two experimental designs have been used to test the effect of the substances suggested by Feingold on hyperactivity: Diet Crossover Studies and Specific Challenge Experiments.

DIET CROSSOVER STUDIES

In a Diet Crossover Study, the scientist selects groups of hyperactive children and places them on two different experimental diets for a specific time period, usually several weeks. One diet follows Dr. Feingold's recommendations; the other is disguised to look like Feingold's but actually contains salicylates, artificial colors and flavors. The behavior of the children is observed and tested while they are on both diets. If behavior is less hyperactive on the Feingold diet, his theory would be supported.

Parents, teachers, and trained observers were all instructed to watch the children's behavior and record their observations. In several experiments, tests of learning ability and other psychological functions thought to measure hyperactivity were also included.

Several Diet Crossover Studies have been completed, but the findings have not been consistent. Some children appeared to improve on the Feingold diet, while others showed no change or worsened. In many cases there were differences in the assessments of the same child's behavior among the different observers and tests. When the data from all the Diet Crossover Studies were compiled, it became evident that parents *frequently* reported an improvement, teachers *sometimes* reported a change, and *no* outside observer reported a reduction in hyperactivity when the child was on the Feingold diet. When additional learning and psychological tests were conducted, these measures did not reflect a behavioral change when the child was on the diet without salicylates, artificial colors and flavors.

The results of the Diet Crossover Studies give little support to the Feingold hypothesis but do not conclusively refute it. When scientists began to analyze the diet therapy more closely, they realized that Dr. Feingold's recommendations caused important changes in family life-style that could also affect the hyperactive child's behavior. Thus, when a reduction in hyperactivity *was* observed in a Diet Crossover Study, it was impossible to pinpoint which of these different changes had caused the improvement.

Because of these problems, conclusions about the Feingold diet could not be made on the basis of Diet Crossover Studies alone, so a second type of study, with a design that permitted scientists to attribute any observed behavioral change to artificial food colors, was carried out.

SPECIFIC CHALLENGE EXPERIMENTS

In a Specific Challenge Experiment, a group of children appearing to respond to the Feingold diet with a reduction in hyperactivity is selected. The children are divided into a test group and a control group. Usually there is also a second testing period in which the group assignments are reversed, so that each child can act as his own control.

Both groups of children are fed a diet free of salicylates, artificial colors, and flavors. The test group is also fed a food that appears to meet the Feingold diet guidelines but that actually contains artificial food colors. The control group is fed a food similar in every way but that does not contain the additives. The behavior of both groups is observed, tested, and compared.

At the time of this writing, seven of these studies have been carried out. Four research teams fed the children in their groups a quantity of an artificial food color blend estimated to be about the average daily consumption of an American child. They divided this quantity in half and fed it in two doses hidden in the special food "treats." A fifth research team fed a specially formulated soft drink containing a quantity of artificial food colors that was slightly greater than the amount used in the two food treats. The sixth study used almost four times this amount, a quantity of artificial food colors considerably greater than the daily consumption of most American children. The seventh experiment used only tartrazine, Yellow Dye #5.

In the study using the large amount of food colors, scores on a learning test declined slightly after the additives were eaten. The group of children fed Yellow Dye #5 showed no change in hyperactivity after the food color was consumed.

Of the five research teams which used the quantity of food colors estimated to be a child's average daily consumption, two found a small but statistically significant increase in hyperactivity after the additives were eaten. Three groups, however, found that the additives had no effect on behavior.

IS THERE A RELATIONSHIP?

These experiments, despite their inconsistent results, do prove that salicylates, artificial colors and flavors *do not* have the dramatic impact on hyperactivity that Dr. Feingold predicted. If artificial colors and flavors are related to behavior, the relationship must be a rather insignificant one. The evidence seems to indicate that a few hyperkinetic children, a fraction of 1 percent, *may* experience a mild adverse reaction to one or several of the artificial colors and flavors in our food supply.

In light of this evidence, Dr. Feingold's reports of a dramatic improvement in patients on his diet must be closely scrutinized. He did not consider what effects the parents' highly emotional response to his diet therapy might have on their perception of their child's hyperactive symptoms, or what impact this enthusiasm might have on the actual behavior of the child. Dr. Feingold attributed all observed behavioral changes to the substances eliminated from the diet and failed to note the possible effect on hyperactivity of other circumstances in the child's life, which also change when his therapy is closely followed.

When the data from the Diet Crossover Studies and Specific Challenge Experiments are compared, they indicate that the changes in family dynamics that occur when the Feingold regimen is strictly followed seem to produce an improvement in the behavior of some hyperactive children. Because it does no physical harm, it would appear that the diet regimen might be helpful therapy in some instances because of its impact on the family. The potential benefits, however, must be weighed against the potentially harmful, long-term educational impact of communicating to a child that his behavior is controlled by what he eats, when in fact this is not true.

Hyperactivity will continue to be a frustrating problem until research resolves the questions of its cause, or causes, and develops an effective treatment. The reality is that we still have a great deal to learn about this condition. We do know now, however, that the Feingold diet is not the answer. It is clear that the symptoms of the vast majority of children labeled "hyperactive" are not related to salicylates, artificial food colors, or artificial flavors. The Feingold diet creates extra work for the homemaker and changes the family life-style . . . but it doesn't cure hyperactivity.

Childhood Behavior and Dr. Lendon Smith

One of the most devastating food books of all time is Dr. Lendon Smith's *Feed Your Kids Right,* published in 1979. Smith has surefire cures for every complaint of childhood by manipulating the diet and megadosing with vitamins and/or minerals.

An Oregon pediatrician for many years, Dr. Smith really

ought to have more sense. Or so we originally thought until we learned that his license to practice medicine had been revoked in 1973 by the Board of Medical Examiners of the state of Oregon. The order of revocation reads in part:

> That the licentiate failed to comply with the standards and conduct of a person of his medical training and education in the City of Portland, State of Oregon, in that he failed to treat the following patients of his in the manner required of a person of his training and education in the field of medicine in the City of Portland, in the manner indicated and as set forth below at the time and dates as specified;
>
> That the licentiate knew it was not necessary to treat the patients listed hereinafter in this manner in order to restore the patient to his health; that the amount and type of drugs the said licentiate was prescribing for the patients listed below was not necessary or medically indicated.

After a series of modifications of the original order, Smith's license was eventually restored, *except* that he remains under certain restrictions in prescribing drugs. This hardly sounds like someone to whom parents should be entrusting their children's health, but his popularity continues. He still frequently delivers speeches and appears on talk shows. As in matters of weight reduction, a gullible public is eager to believe there is an easy way to raise children.

Some of the gems culled from Smith's book are truly preposterous:

> If your child is to have surgery, bring some protein snack to the operating room—not for you, but for the surgeon.

> A poor sense of humor may be the first clue of a vitamin B_3 (niacin) deficiency.

> When your children tire of raw vegetables, whole-wheat bread, nuts, fruits, and salads and ask you, "When are you going to have something good?" tell them, "I would love to give you junk, but I'm afraid you might die of appendicitis, like Aunt Ellie."

I asked a twelve-year-old boy picked up for stealing a television set from a home what he had eaten on the day he did the theft. The only thing he had eaten was a bowl of processed cereal with sugar at eight-thirty in the morning. The crime occurred at 4:30 P.M. The circuits in his conscience that store the message, "Do not steal," were out, and his internal social controls were nonoperative.

I am impressed by how many of these young people show an abnormal glucose tolerance. Because they are eating so poorly, they don't know what they are doing.

The book is filled with similar messages. Throughout, readers are warned to avoid what Smith terms "antinutrients": refined sugar, excessive carbohydrates, and artificial additives. Packaged cereals and white-flour products are also anathema. "Bugs avoid white bread," says Smith. (That may depend on how hungry the bug is, but, to our knowledge, bugs-in-the-bread has never presented a major kitchen dilemma.)

Smith also suggests eating natural foods four to six times a day and advises a basic collection of dietary supplements—in over-ample doses, of course. But that's just for starters. For specific disorders, his recommendations and warnings run the gamut from silly to ludicrous.

A few samples:

- Anxiety is aggravated by low blood sugar and requires megadoses of vitamins A, B_6, C, and pantothenic acid.
- Bed-wetting may be helped by magnesium supplements.
- Autism may be due to zinc deficiency.
- Juvenile delinquency is caused by sugar and white-flour products.
- Depression is linked to low blood sugar and requires extra B vitamins and zinc.
- Psychoses may be caused by copper from copper tubing in the water supply.
- Insomnia can be cured with B vitamins, calcium, and magnesium.

- Irritability is relieved by megadoses of vitamin C.
- Lying is caused by low blood sugar.
- Memory can be improved by additional vitamin B_6.
- Tics can be overcome with massive doses of vitamins C, B complex, B_6 (listed separately, though it is part of the B complex), pantothenic acid (another B vitamin), and calcium (in the form of dolomite, bone meal, or a calcium salt). In addition, Smith advocates nibbling "nutritious" foods every two to three hours to "maintain blood sugar as evenly as possible."

Smith proposes similar remedies for virtually every other kind of malady of childhood: fainting, headbanging, fears, exhaustion, vandalism, dyslexia, and headaches. The entire concept seems much like the faulty notion of reviving a balky car engine by dumping into it as much gasoline, oil, and battery acid it can hold.

The sword is double-edged. There will be those parents who actually take Smith's book seriously and load up their children with supplements that are either useless or potentially harmful. But equally damaging—perhaps more so—are those parents who will choose to rely on dietary supplements as a substitute for personal attention. Instead of working with their children to straighten out the inevitable kinks, to teach them proper behavior, to listen to them, have fun with them, and offer emotional support when needed, how much easier it is to haul out the vitamins and minerals and take away the sugar.

Then when Johnny or Jenny exhibits antisocial behavior or shows evidence of psychological disturbances, it is a simple matter to blame it on the possibility that he or she ate the wrong type of bread (the kind with no bugs in it) in the school lunchroom. The prospect is not only alarming, it is revolting.

In a recent review of *Feed Your Kids Right,* Dr. Manfred Kroger, professor of Food Science at Pennsylvania State University, has stated with great restraint: "I . . . feel that it is imprudent and unreasonable to endorse this book. I wholeheartedly do not recommend it."

Hypoglycemia and Crime

A Washington attorney by the name of Blaine Friedlander believes 80 percent of all juvenile offenders have hypoglycemia (low blood sugar). His theory is not based on careful laboratory testing; it is merely derived from a simple checklist of symptoms that is filled out for each client. (We have already noted at length in chapter 7 that hypoglycemia is actually a rare disorder and that regular periodic drops in blood sugar are perfectly normal.)

Barbara Reed, a probation officer in Ohio, also cites hypoglycemia, together with other forms of "poor nutrition," as a cause of crime. And proponents of orthomolecular psychiatry, the megadosing treatment described in the last chapter, attribute criminal behavior to low blood sugar, deficiency of vitamins B_6 and B_{12}, plus an excessive intake of caffeine.

Those are only a few examples of what is happening in certain areas of our judicial system. Noticeably absent in such defense of criminals, however, is any mention of the health status of their victims.

Sugar and Behavior Problems

Carrying this lack of logic a step further is the contention that consumption of sugar and sugar products in itself causes deviant behavior—with or without hypoglycemia. In 1978, after killing the mayor of San Francisco, Dan White's legal defense was based in part on the fact that he had eaten a lot of junk food shortly before the murder (this has been described as the so-called "Twinkie" defense). And after the death of Sharon Tate in the late sixties, Adelle Davis enjoyed sharing her opinion that the infamous Manson "family" had committed the murder because they had been subsisting for days on candy bars. "Where the diet is good," she once declared, "there is no crime."

The odds aren't too good here. Billions of people eat sugar

products every day—have done so for years—and *don't* commit murder. They don't steal television sets; they don't attack their next-door neighbors; they don't destroy public schools.

The idea that some persons might be "allergic" to sugar is likewise illogical. The end product of sugar metabolism is glucose, the same as it is from all other forms of carbohydrates, including starches. Carbohydrates must be in the form of glucose to be used by the body, which doesn't know, and couldn't care less, where its glucose supply originated.

We are perfectly aware that poor eating habits are frequently part of a generally poor environment that sometimes contributes to criminal behavior. But it is not sugar alone—or any other substance, or the lack of any substance—that creates a criminal. Like an alcoholic blaming his liver problems on white bread or food coloring, sugar is but an easy mark. The hypothesis is totally devoid of sense or scientific fact.

Nutritional Cures for Depression

Serotonin, a neurotransmitter essential to proper brain function, is a favorite topic among serious health faddists. According to articles in *Prevention* magazine, low levels of serotonin also cause depression. We are then informed—and this part is scientific fact—that tryptophan, an essential amino acid, is needed to produce serotonin.

Then, in typical misstatement of facts, the reader is told that vitamin B_6 is needed to produce tryptophan; thus, depressed people need more B_6. This is blatant misinformation. Tryptophan, like all essential amino acids, cannot be synthesized by the body. That is why amino acids are called "essential"; we have to get them from the foods we eat. No amount of vitamin B_6 will produce more tryptophan than we ingest in the form of protein.

The only connection between tryptophan and vitamin B_6 is that in the presence of B_6 plus thiamine and riboflavin, tryptophan can be converted to niacin if the body needs it. (And here we remind you again that niacin is now practically never deficient in this country.) If the last two paragraphs have been difficult to follow, we urge you to reread them, because they constitute a perfect example of the distortions offered so ubiquitously by the health-food faddists.

Of course, there are any number of other "cures" for depression. If vitamin B_6 doesn't do the trick, you can try straight niacin. And if that doesn't work, try calcium, or magnesium, "the natural sedative." Last, but not least, if all else fails, say the hoaxsters, you can be reasonably sure if you're still depressed that you have low blood sugar. Or that salt is holding water in the tissues (which it does) and creating pressure on your brain. (There is no evidence supporting the latter.)

However, during the course of attempting this entire string of remedies, we sincerely hope that the real underlying cause or causes of the depression have abated. Severe depression usually requires some form of professional help. If the condition is neglected in favor of useless vitamin/mineral or similar treatment, it could evolve into a major psychological disturbance.

Aphrodisiacs

Throughout history love potions have been highly sought-after commodities. One of the longest lived is a mixture of fish roe and wine that was first popular among the ancient Greeks. There are those who still consider this combination effective, although today the items are served separately, preferably by candlelight, in the form of caviar and champagne.

At one time or another, aphrodisiac qualities have probably been attributed to almost every conceivable substance on earth. In the past there were rhinoceros horn, dried salamander, walnuts, radishes, and parsley, but our modern generation is more likely to be found experimenting with ginseng root and vitamin E.

There is no evidence whatever that any food has ever actually functioned as an aphrodisiac or that it has enhanced anyone's sex appeal. However, to quote Richard R. Mathison in *The Eter-*

nal Search: "Authorities agree . . . that if a man believes that potato parings or crocodile steak will make him virile, it often will, for the state of the psychic and spiritual being casts a long shadow over man's sexual doings."

The same principle can be applied to any substance consumed for any other purpose. The will to believe can sometimes accomplish wonders.

Conclusions

The time has come for people to resume responsibility for their own actions—and to help their children do the same. Youngsters raised under the misconception that food is in some way responsible for their behavior are being treated unfairly. Inevitably, they will sooner or later encounter a rude awakening.

In the presence of true sensitivity to certain foods (really quite rare) or diet-related diseases or disorders, diet modification under professional care is necessary. For the vast majority of the healthy population, however, a balanced diet will supply all needed nutrients—independent of what kinds of carbohydrate are included or what color the flour is. At best, megadosing with dietary supplements may provide a temporary placebo effect; at worst, the practice may be disastrous.

Man is not a slave to dietary indiscretions. Sugar doesn't incite him to rob a bank; food additives do not make a child quarrelsome; phosphorus does not endow one with superintelligence. Good general eating habits, along with other good health habits, promote a sound body and a sound mind. But no single substance, or its lack, directly affects one's moral judgments in either thought or action.

> It's a very odd thing—
> As odd as can be—
> That whatever Miss T eats
> Turns into Miss T.
>
> —WALTER DE LA MARE

CHAPTER 10

Nutrition Information: Whom Do You Believe?

IF YOU HAVE READ THIS FAR IN THE BOOK, you must surely be aware that the declarations of the health quacks are simply not all they're cracked up to be. Nevertheless, perhaps you still have reservations.

"But vitamins make me *feel* better," we are sometimes told. "And brewer's yeast did wonders for Aunt Hattie."

What is often at work here is commonly known as the placebo effect: If you *think* a useless substance is going to work, it often will—like the child who insists his bruised finger doesn't hurt as much with a Band-Aid on it. Ignoring minor complaints often results in their disappearance.

The converse is also true. If we *look* for a symptom, it is often very easy to find. If someone you believe in tells you that sugar will make you sluggish and you have just eaten a sweet dessert for lunch, you may very well end up with a case of the blahs in the afternoon. The feeling may result from too much total lunch, or the weather, or an unpleasant encounter with a co-worker, or it might have passed entirely unnoticed if you hadn't been watching for it. (In any case, sugar—an energy food—does *not* cause sluggishness.) If you are truly convinced of the relationship, you may rush to tell all your friends, thus perpetuating another myth.

Similarly, in the absence of controlled scientific conditions, there is no way to prove—or disprove—that any disorder did not disappear of its own accord. Vitamin A supplements might *seem* to have cured a teenager's acne, but more than likely the time was right for it to clear up anyway.

Suggestion is a very powerful force. The interplay of mind and body is not yet well understood by psychiatrists or other medical doctors or scientists; they do know, however, that it exists. If you firmly believe that vitamins or other dietary supplements make you "feel better," then *in moderate amounts* they probably constitute a safer psychological crutch than many other substances. If you honestly prefer organically grown foods and can afford them, they are unlikely to cause any harm. But if you are on a tight budget, you should be aware that none of these foods or supplements is necessary for good health—and that the claims made for them are generally unsupported by scientific fact.

Business vs. Business

A number of health frauds have attempted to impress the public with the peculiar dichotomy that every spokesperson for health must be either "consumer-oriented" or "industry-oriented." That's very much like saying that food processors are not a part of the consumer market, and that health-food stores are nonprofit institutions.

It is a mistake to assume that the health-food industry is entirely pro-consumer, and that those defending other food systems are not. Surely it is obvious that everyone must eat, including food manufacturers and all the farmers who rely on traditional agricultural methods. And certainly it must be equally apparent that we all wish to remain healthy. It is also foolish to suppose that members of the health-food, ordinary food, and pharmaceutical industries are not in their respective businesses to make money.

In essence, then, the issue becomes one of pitting one businessman against another. But in this case, it is not one of healthy competition. (Rather, it may be *un*healthy in every sense of the word.) Misinformation, and often vicious propaganda, are advanced against the traditional food industry and its defenders by those affiliated with the health-food industry. At the same time, their own contentions are promoted by the use of a smattering of facts mixed with a great deal of blarney and unsubstantiated testimonials.

We would be naive as well as incorrect to suggest that one side is always all "good" and the other all "bad." The health foodists' rejection of facts, as well as their inconsistent accusations, do not constitute a sensible philosophy. Those of us who approach questions about sugar, food additives, and processing from an appropriate scientific perspective are often dismissed as "hired guns"—frequently when there is no connection whatever with any branch of industry. Yet a quack on the payroll of, say, a vitamin company is acceptable, apparently because vitamins are acceptable. But if a legitimate scientist then issues a warning against megadosing, from ocean to ocean the cry is heard: "Spokesman for industry!"

Carlton Fredericks is a regular columnist for *Prevention* magazine. *Prevention* is filled with articles and columns advocating the need for food supplements, and its pages carry an amazing collection of ads for those same supplements. The connection here is obvious—but it is ignored by the anti-industry health messiahs.

The conclusion is simple: To health-foodists, truth is both unprofitable and ego-damaging.

What Is a Nutritionist?

Nutrition is big business, and the field is open to everyone. In medicine and most other health professional fields, educational standards are controlled by laws which protect the public. There are regulations that determine who may call themselves physicians, dentists, nurses, and pharmacists, for instance. But this is not true in nutrition. Anyone who so chooses can designate himself or herself a nutrition "expert" or "nutritionist."

What training do nutritionists receive? Some hold legitimate health credentials. Others have mail-order degrees or no training at all. Worthless credentials may often resemble valuable ones. How can the consumer tell the difference?

Betsy McPherrin, a nutrition researcher for the American Council on Science and Health, suggests that an individual who consults a nutritionist should look for specific professional credentials; academic degrees from accredited institutions, membership in the major professional societies, board certification, or registration in dietetics.

Training in nutrition at accredited universities provides a sound scientific background. Unfortunately, many small unaccredited correspondence schools also offer degrees in nutrition. To see if your nutritionist's degree represents real scientific training, check to see if the college that issued it is accredited. Unaccredited schools often have incomplete or questionable progams that differ greatly from those of respected universities.

Those nutrition specialists who hold doctoral degrees can seek certification—another guarantee that the nutritionist's credentials are sound. The American Board of Nutrition certifies M.D.'s as specialists in clinical nutrition, and both M.D.'s and Ph.D.'s as specialists in human nutritional sciences. Board-certified nutrition specialists must pass a comprehensive examination on all phases of nutrition, including deficiency disease, metabolism, food/drug interaction, therapeutic diets, and the derivation and use of the recommended dietary allowances for essential nutrients.

Nutritionists at the doctoral level may also be members of two prestigious professional organizations, both of which have stringent requirements for membership: the American Institute of Nutrition (AIN) and the American Society for Clinical Nutrition (ASCN).

Another type of qualified nutritionist is the registered dietitian (R.D.), who is specially trained to translate nutrition research into healthful, tasty diets. Registered dietitians hold bachelor's or master's degrees in nutrition and must have professional experience and take a comprehensive written examination before qualifying for R.D. certification.

Ms. McPherrin warns that unqualified nutritionists, realizing the value of professional achievement, may also display credentials that appear as impressive as the legitimate credentials described above. Degrees from unaccredited schools are one example. Another is ANCA (American Nutritional Consultants Association) membership. Unlike AIN or ASCN, membership in this organization is not a matter of professional achievement. For a twenty-five dollar fee, anyone can buy membership in ANCA and thus be entitled to use the initials after his or her name.

The N.D. (Doctor of Naturopathy) degree displayed by many popular self-styled "nutritionists" may be obtained by correspondence course and encompasses unorthodox treatment methods such as homeopathy, reflexology, biofeedback and autogenic training, joint and muscle manipulation, dietary supplements, herbalism, spinal manipulation, and acupuncture. Recently we noticed a new twist on "naturopathy." An advertisement in the back of a health-food magazine announced the availability of mail-order courses in "nutripathy."

The initials C.H. stand for "certified herbologist," D.C. for "doctor of chiropractic," R.H. for "registered healthologist," C.A. for "certified acupuncturist." None of these signify competence in nutrition, but they are often used and displayed by self-styled nutritionists.

Organizations often cited in the biographical data of would-be nutritionists include the International Academy of Biological Medicine, the International Naturopathic Association, the International Society for Research on Civilization Diseases and Environment, the Academy of Orthomolecular Psychiatry, the International Academy of Preventive Medicine, the American Academy of Medical Preventics, and the Orthomolecular Medical Society.

These seemingly professional "credentials" are undeservingly worth both money and respect. In some fields of endeavor, phony credentials have little effect on the public. Unfortunately, this is not so with nutrition, a field with serious health implications. If you consult a nutritionist, it would be prudent to check his/her credentials thoroughly.

See Your Doctor

One of your best sources of reliable nutrition information is a person whom few people consider a diet authority—your family doctor.

A lot of people have made a big fuss over physicians' supposedly inadequate knowledge of nutrition. But, in fact, doctors know a great deal about this subject as a result of the biochemical and physiological training they received in medical school. They also know enough science to be able to separate nutrition fact from nutrition fiction. Both responsible and fraudulent nutrition information may contain a lot of biochemical details unfamiliar to most of us. It is difficult for most people to tell if they are confronting sound chemical science or chemical gibberish. Your physician can help you to make this distinction. He or she has enough scientific training to determine rather quickly whether a popular diet book is based on facts or misinformation, and to conclude whether a "new nutritional discovery" is a real scientific development or a piece of quack nonsense.

Unfortunately, a few physicians have gotten caught up in nutrition misinformation. Some practice scientifically questionable "orthomolecular medicine," and a few have even written unsound fad-diet books. But the vast majority of physicians have nothing to do with these fringe practices. Don't overlook your family doctor as a good source of reliable, believable advice about nutrition.

Whelan/Stare Lawsuit

In December 1978 the two of us became the target of a libel suit filed by the National Nutritional Foods Association (NNFA), a health-food trade group, in addition to David T. Ajay, owner of Dave's Diet and Nutrition Foods in Sacramento, California; Sid Cammy, owner of The Diet Shop in Elizabeth, New Jersey; and Max Huberman, owner of Natural Health Foods in Youngstown, Ohio. The plaintiffs were asking for $1.3 million in damages, allegedly resulting from our "conspiracy to defame, disparage, damage, and destroy [their] reputation and business." Among those named as co-conspirators in the suit were columnist Ann Landers; Dr. Philip White of the American Medical Association; and Dr. William T. Jarvis of Loma Linda University in Southern California, who is president of the California Council Against Health Fraud.

The complaint alleged that statements we had made questioning the health benefits of foods labeled "organic" or "natural" had led to a decline in sales of such products, and that we had "acted in a malicious, willful and grossly irresponsible manner" in publishing these remarks in our syndicated newspaper column, "Food and Your Health," as well as in an article in *Harper's Bazaar* and in our 1975 book, *Panic in the Pantry.*

Since none of these publications mentioned any of the individual plaintiffs or their businesses, we answered in part that NNFA's action "must be viewed as an effort, under the guise of an alleged defamation suit, to stifle public criticism." At no time were we alarmed by the accusations; we knew that we had more than enough evidence to back up all we had said, and we were willing to fight. To us, the lawsuit constituted living proof that the health-food industry does indeed have the truth to fear.

The libel suit was dismissed a year and a half later (on June 21, 1980) by the U.S. District Court of New York Southern District.* A libel claim requires proof of false statements. Judge Abraham D. Sofaer found that "each of the opinions expressed by the defendants about the health-food industry has sufficient basis in fact or responsible opinion to make it impossible to believe that plaintiffs could prove falsity."

The judge further stated that, in his opinion "misuse of the term 'organic' has been widely condemned," that "health-food-store prices have been shown to be often higher than prices for comparable products in other food stores," and that "persons advocating or selling health-food items have been found to give improper health advice, amounting to 'quackery,' and to make unsupportable claims for health products and vitamins." Moreover, the court stated that *"the public's gain from activities such as those engaged in by defendants clearly outweighs the harm to groups and individuals such as plaintiffs."*

EVEN WHEN YOU WIN, YOU LOSE A LITTLE

The cost of legal defense in a suit of these proportions is exceedingly high. In addition, there is an enormous amount of time required in preparing the defense, and there is disruption of other work. Leonard J. Theberge, executive director of The Media Institute, has put it very well: "A libel lawsuit can be a powerful weapon to silence the expression of unwanted facts and opinions. While the plaintiff is put through the legal expense of preparing and filing a complaint, the financial burden shifts immediately to the defendant. Moreover, a defendant is effectively prevented from commenting on the subject matter during the lawsuit and must, in preparing his defense, turn his attention away from research and the expression of critical views."

* Our legal counselor in this matter was Robert Stitt, Esq., a partner in the New York law firm Thacher Proffitt and Wood.

It is for precisely those reasons that similar lawsuits in the past have caused defendants to knuckle under. A case in point is that of John F. Duffy, sheriff of California's San Diego County, who has also been the subject of NNFA legal action.

Because he was concerned about the popularity of what Duffy described as "different forms of health quackery" among the senior citizens in his jurisdiction, the sheriff began to distribute, as a public service, an educational booklet entitled, "Beware Health 'Quackery.' " The NNFA, in a letter signed by David Ajay dated August 7, 1978, requested Duffy to withdraw the booklet from circulation. When the sheriff refused, the trade association filed suit against him in San Diego Superior Court that October.

To date, there have been no further proceedings in the case—possibly because the printers of the sheriff's pamphlet, after communication with the NNFA, withdrew the booklet from further publication.

This kind of harassment is nothing short of blackmail.

In our own case, we were indeed fortunate to receive immediate financial support from a great many scientists and other responsible citizens who were thoroughly disgusted with NNFA's attempts to manipulate the public and who wanted the truth laid before the public. Without such assistance we, too, might have been forced to back away.

During the course of our lawsuit, a *Wall Street Journal* editorial about it noted: "The suit doesn't look like a winner, but such attempts at intimidation have considerable harassment value. . . . Attacking the establishment nowadays is a pretty fair way to make a living; defending it, it seems, is only going to get you hauled into court."

THE ACCUSERS WAIL

Our recent libel suit was not the first time we had met with adversity. One of us (FJS) has been criticized frequently over the years as a "pawn" of industry, particularly in relation to sugar and breakfast cereals. The facts simply do not bear out any of the accusations.

Not once during FJS's thirty-four years as chairman of Harvard's Department of Nutrition was a single industry or other private grant accepted for work on a specific industrial product or problem. The only restrictions whatever came from government grants and contracts, where policy dictates that funds be delegated only for specific purposes. During the first twenty years of the department's existence (1942–62), unrestricted grants were received from 47 companies, 10 trade associations, 18 foundations, 3 national voluntary health agencies, as well as 138 grants from the National Institutes of Health, 13 grants or contracts from other federal agencies, and funds from 76 private individuals.

Although sugar has endured as a prime focus, the first funding from any company or trade association in the sugar industry was not granted until the 1961–62 year and, as with all other grants, was completely unrestricted. Furthermore, FJS's publicly stated scientific information about sugar predates that occasion by many years.

The Nutrition Research Laboratories at Harvard, completed in the early sixties, cost just over $5 million. Of this sum, approximately 25 percent came from the food industry, about twice that amount from foundations and various individuals, and the balance from the National Institutes of Health. Despite this carefully documented and easily accessible information, at least one of CBS' "60 Minutes" programs blatantly led its viewers to believe otherwise.

As far back as 1959, FJS was sued by the Boston Nutrition Society for an answer he had prepared to a question received from the editorial staff of *McCall's* magazine. His response had appeared in the March 1957 issue as part of a question-and-answer column and concerned the veracity of a Boston Nutrition Society claim that white bread was devoid of nutrients and related to the development of both heart disease and cancer. FJS wrote: "To imply or suggest that enriched white bread can cause or contribute to diseases listed in the clipping is a cruel and reckless fraud."

The case was first heard before a Massachusetts Superior Court and dismissed. The plaintiffs then appealed to the Supreme Judicial Court of Massachusetts, which ordered the case to be submitted to a jury. After four days of testimony in 1962, the jury deliberated only fifteen minutes and acquitted FJS.

In the years since, the charges and threats have been various and numerous. In the absence of any real basis for complaint, the accusers must resort to the cry of "Tainted money!"

This is nonsense. The fact is that any university receives its funding from many sources, private and government, as well as industry. There is no reason to believe that anyone trained in the scientific method is going to be influenced by the source of payment for his or her scientific endeavors. There are undoubtedly a few exceptions—just as there are a few physicians who appear to have departed from reason in their unorthodox methods of treatment.

Similarly, when the Food and Nutrition Board of the National Academy of Sciences took a position on the relationship of dietary fat and cholesterol to heart disease that appeared to differ from the positions of some other prominent organizations, it encountered considerable controversy. The opposition attempted to tie the new recommendations to the food industry by noting that various members of the board had food-industry connections and some had received monies from food companies, either directly as fees for consultation or indirectly as research grants through their respective institutions. It is simplistic to assume that judgment is distorted or integrity soiled merely because one is, or has been, a paid consultant. There is no good reason to forego funding assistance from credible corporations and foundations which bestow grants for the purpose of establishing and maintaining the type of scientific and educational research that ultimately serves the common welfare of American consumers.

A certain amount of contact with industry is desirable in order to understand many of the problems of society and help to solve them. What may seem feasible within the confines of a laboratory or under the protective shroud of academia does not necessarily afford a workable solution in the real world. The majority, if not all, of the food industry is indeed striving continually to improve its products. The notion that it is spending its research dollars to achieve the opposite is totally devoid of logic.

A TURNING POINT

Although we were not awarded legal fees for our recent libel suit on the grounds that there was no firm evidence that the plaintiffs had acted in bad faith, the court warned that "any further suit by plaintiffs against critics of the health-food industry should, however, be scrutinized carefully to determine whether it was brought in good faith." Perhaps our efforts have served to hinder the health-foodists in their war against truth.

R. L. Hall, past president of the Institute of Food Technologists, has commented: "The flow and counterflow of ideas is an essential part of the scientific process. Everywhere scientists gather, ideas are put forward, rebutted, modified, and tested again. False or inadequate information is thus corrected, expanded, or clarified, and gradually a more accurate picture of our surroundings appears. When such corrective procedures are hindered, serious misinformation can be promulgated, leading to incorrect decision and even to actual harm to individuals and to society."

And Harry G. Day, professor emeritus of chemistry at Indiana University in Bloomington, stated: "The effrontery of the National Nutritional Foods Association in bringing suit against F. J. Stare and E. M. Whelan should galvanize determined action across the entire country to combat such misuse of the courts, and it should stimulate a strong reaction against the use of half-truths and extravagant advertising to exploit credulous and uninformed people. Let every trained and responsible nutritionist become personally committed to actively challenging intimidation and quackery in every form."

Hope glimmers on the horizon.

Popularity vs. Truth

We are only too keenly aware that we do not find ourselves on the most popular side of the entire food issue. Our fan mail is not always the kind we like to receive. From all points of the globe letters arrive, flatly declaring us "wrong" about some point or other, and rarely do they offer any source for their "information." Those that do, almost without exception, merely parrot advice from the quacks or refer to a study that has never been validated (although it may have been well publicized).

Critics of science find a difficult task dealing with facts; there simply isn't enough evidence on which to base their contentions. Thus, when we recently challenged the Feingold Association (of hyperkinesis fame), its only recourse was to make loud noises about funding.

Ours Is Not the Final Word

We do not expect you to agree with everything we have said. Rarely are even any two scientists in 100 percent agreement in all matters of interpretation. By the time this book goes to press, it is highly possible new evidence will have been amassed that may modify our own thinking in certain areas.

Basically, what we are recommending is that for your own protection you keep an open mind. Listen to all viewpoints and weigh them carefully. Consider the credentials and motivations of those involved.

THE MISINFORMATION INFLATION

We are not suggesting that it is a simple task to decide what—or whom—to believe. Misinformation can be presented most convincingly, as one quack quotes another and alludes to him or her as a "great scientist." They mix together valid and invalid studies, good and poor reasoning, scientific data with nonsense, and refer vaguely to "published studies" (both their own and those of the other "great scientists").

When Adelle Davis warned that we had the Russians to fear because they eat much less of the "illness-breeding refined foods" than do Americans, it is difficult to believe that anyone could have taken her seriously—but someone probably did. (The assertion was no worse, however, than her suggestion that the reason Germany defeated France in World War II was because German black bread and beer are nutritionally superior to French white bread and wine.)

Further, we wish to caution against making premature assumptions. One or two quick studies prove nothing, however appealing the proposed theory might be to scientists and nonscientists alike. Sound scientific principles are based on many years of in-depth study and research.

And whenever you feel unsure of what or whom to believe, you should realize that it is far better to err on the side of conservatism. The nutrition hoax can be life-threatening.

How to Spot a Quack*

Below, we have set forth a few tips to help you recognize the possibility that you are being "taken." Not all the characteristics are usually present in equal degree; some may be expressed quite subtly. But most of them are there most of the time.

(1) The quack *always* has something to sell: a course of lectures, vitamin preparations, tonics, nature foods, diet plans, reducing machines, natural cosmetics, books, spe-

* These tips are adapted from a more extensive discussion of how to spot a quack by Drs. Victor Herbert and Stephen Barrett in their recent book *Vitamins and "Health" Foods: The Great American Hustle* (Philadelphia: George F. Stickley Co., 1981).

cial nutrient-preserving cookware, water purifiers, ad infinitum.

(2) The quack usually claims to be a "medical expert" or a "leading nutritionist," and is often the president or director of an important-sounding (if nonexistent) "scientific society." Like the plaque on the kitchen wall designating the "world's greatest cook," there is nothing illegal in adopting such titles; anyone can do it.

(3) The quack often claims to have some secret formula or knowledge that will cure whatever ails you.

(4) The quack promises a quick cure, on a money-back basis, "if your arthritis isn't cured in eight days," or "if you don't lose ten pounds the first week." If the results do not materialize, he tells you that you didn't follow the instructions correctly—or that yours is a rare case that requires his extra-potency formula (or whatever), which he then proceeds to sell you.

(5) The quack is prone to speak in terms of "subclinical deficiencies"; that is, a deficiency not severe enough to be detectable by ordinary methods. He further suggests that everyone is suffering from poor nutrition.

(6) The quack distorts scientific data to suit his own ends.

(7) Similarly, the quack puts together his own *un*scientific data. He may tell you that diet causes disease, that artificial additives are poisoning the food supply, that chemical fertilizers are causing malnutrition, that the processing of food removes all its nutrients, or all of these. And others.

(8) The quack informs you that even if you eat badly, his special vitamin formula with 217 different nutrients can save your life.

(9) The quack uses testimonials and case histories to "prove" that his product is miraculous. He does *not* offer facts based on carefully controlled studies, published in reputable medical journals and confirmed by independent workers.

(10) The quack claims to be persecuted by scientists and/or government agencies because, he insists, the medical profession and the Food and Drug Administration are corrupt and influenced solely by big business.

Recommendations

The bottom line is that it's *your* health we're talking about: Don't squander either it or your money. You have the right to be as suspicious and hypercritical as you wish.

There are some mistakes you can't afford to make.

CHAPTER 11

What Is Good Nutrition?

SO FAR, WE HAVE BEEN WRITING MOSTLY about nutrition hoaxes, what we frequently refer to as "nutrition nonsense." We want to end this book on a positive note. What is good nutrition? What is good diet? What foods should we eat?

The food one eats is a very personal matter. Normally, most people resist following a diet outlined completely and specifically by someone else. The complaints about food that are so often heard in college dormitories and other institutional settings illustrate the emotional value people place upon selecting what they eat.

A menu planned for a sizable group of people may be nutritionally adequate in every way, yet fail to allow for the fact that one or more of the included foods may not be eaten for cultural or personal reasons. Food that is planned but not eaten cannot contribute to good nutrition.

How to Select a Balanced Diet

Clearly, a few guidelines are helpful in planning the daily food intake for you and your family. So that such guides may be more

288

meaningful, we also include here some brief background information.

THE COMPOSITION OF FOOD

The major components in the foods we eat—paralleling our basic nutritional requirements—are protein, fat, carbohydrate, vitamins, minerals, and water. Fiber is sometimes also included, but it consists largely of indigestible carbohydrate, and many nutritionists question whether it can actually be termed an essential nutrient. Fiber does contribute mechanically to good digestion, however, and for that reason alone is highly desirable in the diet.

Only protein, fat, and carbohydrate (and alcohol) provide calories; that is, energy. But they can be utilized only in conjunction with other dietary components. Eating a balanced variety of foods will supply all of the fifty or so known nutrients. The precise number is still in question because the nutritional roles of some substances are not yet fully understood. This is particularly true for some of the trace minerals.

Protein. Proteins are large nitrogen-containing molecules which build and repair tissues and can also furnish energy. The building blocks of proteins are amino acids, of which some twenty are commonly found in nature. Amino acids are formed when protein is broken down in the body; that is, digested. These smaller molecules, amino acids, are carried by the blood to the cells of the body, where they are assembled into body protein, hormones, enzymes and used for different functions.

The nutritional quality of the protein contained in each food depends on its amino acid composition. There are eight essential amino acids, which the adult human body cannot manufacture and which must be obtained from food. The infant and young child require one or two more essential amino acids. Those proteins which contain the essential amino acids in the proportions and the amounts needed by the body for tissue replacement and growth are called "complete" proteins, or proteins with "high biological value." Eggs, milk, meat, fish, cheese, and poultry are examples of such complete protein foods.

On the other hand, some foods lack one or more of the essential amino acids in adequate amounts. If a person uses *solely* these foods, the growth needs of tissue will not be met. These proteins are said to be "incomplete" or of "poor biologic value." Generally, the plant proteins, such as in cereals, vegetables, and legumes, are in this group. However, one protein can supplement another by providing the amino acids that are missing in the first. Many Mexican dishes are a good example of mixtures of different proteins which together can make a complete food. For instance, beans and rice contain incomplete proteins that supplement each other. Eaten together, at the same meal, they provide complete protein. Cereal with milk is another common example of the supplementary action of two proteins. In general, a small amount of animal protein will supplement plant proteins, making the total mixture of high biological value.

Proteins also furnish four calories of energy per gram. If the diet contains more protein than the body needs for building and repairing cells, the amino acid molecules can be used as a source of energy or stored in the form of body fat. If the diet does not provide sufficient energy from fats and carbohydrates, protein will be used for energy, rather than for its main function of building and replacing muscle tissues or for making hormones, enzymes, and other body protein components. This is why it is important to eat a balanced diet providing all nutrients in appropriate amounts.

Carbohydrates. Carbohydrate-rich foods are very common and popular throughout the world. There are two main types of carbohydrates: sugars and starches. In many areas of the world, carbohydrates are the main part of the diet. Cereal grains, rice, and potatoes are the major sources of starch. Cane and beets provide most of the sugar in the diet, in the form of sucrose (also known as "cane sugar"). However, corn, which contains starch that can be converted to glucose and fructose, has also become an important source of sugar in the diet. Rice, wheat, and corn are the leading staple foods of the world. One reason for this is that these products can be grown easily, give a large yield of food per acre, and, as a result, are relatively inexpensive. Sugars are also universally popular and are the most efficient source of calories in terms of land usage.

Carbohydrates supply energy. Each gram of carbohydrate supplies about four calories, regardless of whether it is in the form of starch or sugar. Besides providing energy, carbohydrate-rich foods (except for sugar and cassava) are also good sources of protein, some vitamins (especially from the B group), and some minerals.

Carbohydrates are broken down by the body into their component monosaccharides or simple sugars, namely glucose and fructose. Galactose, another simple sugar, is formed when milk sugar, lactose, is digested. These monosaccharides are absorbed by the small intestine, where all nonglucose simple sugars are converted to their final form, glucose. Glucose is the sugar absorbed into the blood (blood sugar refers to glucose). Shortly after a meal, the blood sugar rises and is carried to all body cells.

Fat. Fats (also called lipids) are simple molecules composed of three elements: carbon, hydrogen, and oxygen. When they are digested, they release a little more than twice as much energy as carbohydrates or proteins (nine calories per gram). Because of this high-energy content, excess fat in a diet can easily contribute to obesity.

Fats are composed of fatty acids—saturated and unsaturated. The saturated fatty acids are those to which no hydrogen can be added to the molecule; the unsaturated fatty acids are those which can still take up some hydrogen. The monounsaturated fatty acids have one "double bond" and can absorb two hydrogen atoms; the polyunsaturated fatty acids have two or more double bonds and can absorb four or more hydrogen atoms. The unsaturated fats are usually in liquid form such as oils. The vegetable oils, such as soya, corn or safflower are usually high in polyunsaturated fats. However, by a process known as hydrogenation, hydrogen can be added, making a solid fat and yielding such products as margarine. Foods such as whole milk, cream, ice cream, egg yolk, meats, and butter are relatively high in saturated fatty acids, as are two vegetable oils—coconut and palm.

PUTTING IT ALL TOGETHER

No single food contains sufficient amounts of all needed nutrients. There is no "perfect food," including mother's milk. To be well nourished one must eat a variety of foods, and with some degree of planning. One useful guide extensively employed in the United States is the plan known as the Basic Four Food Groups.

THE "BASIC FOUR"

About forty years ago the U.S. Department of Agriculture devised the "Basic Seven" food groups to demonstrate the variety of foods needed to achieve good nutrition. This plan was a simplification of the earlier "Basic Eleven." But despite this improvement, it eventually became apparent that a system with seven categories still presented more of a challenge than most people could easily handle. Therefore, in 1955, Harvard's Department of Nutrition suggested a daily food guide comprised of only four basic food groups. A year later, the USDA also settled on the same "Basic Four," and this plan was subsequently adopted by most nutrition education groups in the United States.

The Basic Four is a simple device for establishing adequate nutrition on a daily basis. It is not structured to enumerate all foods needed daily. What it does provide is a practical framework for planning meals that during the course of a day will supply all essential nutrients. Neither sugar nor fats and oils are included because these substances mainly provide calories and are rarely lacking in American diets. Alcohol is not included because it generally is not considered a food. However, it *is* a source of calories, and this must be considered by those who consume alcoholic beverages.

A simplified table of recommended servings and a brief discus
sion of the Basic Four Food Groups appears below:

The Basic Four Food Groups

	Recommended Daily Amount
I. *Meat group,* including poultry, fish, eggs, and legumes	2 or more servings
II. *Milk* and milk products	2 servings—adults 3–4 servings—children
III. *Vegetables and Fruits*	4 or more servings
IV. *Breads and Cereals*	4 or more servings

1 serving of meat = 3 oz.
1 serving of milk = 1 cup or 8 oz. of milk
1 serving of vegetables = ½ cup
1 serving of bread, = 1 slice of bread
                 1 oz. of ready-to-eat cereal
                 ½c cooked rice or macaroni

I. The *meat group* also includes poultry, fish, eggs, nuts, and legumes such as dried beans and peas. All of these are rich sources of protein. In addition, these foods supply vitamins of the B complex, including thiamine, riboflavin, niacin, B_6, and B_{12}, plus minerals, particularly iron. Note that the recommended serving of meat is only 3 ounces. This is about half or less of what most adults usually consume.

II. Foods from the second group, *milk and milk products* (which includes cheese, yogurt, and ice cream as well as milk but not butter), supply more calcium per serving than any other food commonly used in the United States. Indeed, it is difficult for the average American to consume enough calcium without the use of milk or cheese. In addition, these foods provide nutritionally complete protein, many of the B vitamins (especially riboflavin), vitamin A (if the milk is whole milk or fortified skim milk), and vitamin D (if it has been added to the milk as it should be). If you use skim milk, dry skim-milk powder, or low-fat milk, be sure to select those labeled as having vitamins A and D added, because when the butterfat is removed from milk, so are the fat-soluble vitamins. Two servings per day from this group are recom-mended for adults; three to four for children and teenagers.

III. Foods in the *vegetable and fruit group* supply many nutrients: vitamin C, vitamin A, folic acid, important amounts of many minerals, carbohydrates, and fiber. Perhaps just as important, these foods also supply the psychological values of texture, color, and variety.

Since under normal conditions vitamin C is not stored in the body, one serving daily of a food rich in this vitamin is recommended, such as citrus fruit or juice, tomato, or cantaloupe. Often it is most convenient to serve this food at breakfast, but it is just as beneficial at any other meal. In addition, a dark green leafy vegetable, dark yellow vegetable, or other vitamin A-rich food should be served at least every other day. A total of four (or more) servings per day is suggested.

IV. *Breads and cereals*—whole grain or enriched—are valuable sources of carbohydrate, protein, riboflavin, niacin, thiamine, and iron. In fact, it is difficult to obtain a sufficient quantity of the latter two nutrients without these foods. Because for many years Americans have tended to prefer white bread, enrichment laws have been enacted in about half the states (the other states adhere to them voluntarily) which require the replacement of some of the important nutrients that are partially removed during the milling of white flour. Both whole grain and enriched grain products are nutritious foods. Many states and many food companies have also expanded their enrichment programs to use enriched flour in the manufacture of other bakery products and of crackers.

Recommended from this group are four servings daily. A serving is approximately equivalent to one slice of bread, one-half cup of cooked cereal, macaroni or other pasta, or one cup of ready-to-eat cereal.

OTHER FOODS

Almost all of us also consume a selection of fats, sugars, spreads, dressings, sauces, gravies, condiments, and other complements to our food. For many, the day's fare is not complete without beverages (alcoholic and otherwise) and snacks or desserts that don't come from the "Basic Four." Indeed, these additions may collectively increase the daily calorie intake by 25 percent or more. (For overenthusiastic eaters, it is usually *much* more.)

The foods we eat must be put into perspective. When the need arises to cut down on the amount you are eating, these "other foods" are the ones to be sacrificed. Foods from the Basic Four should be left intact. (But even here, you will need to keep the portions small and skip the "seconds" if you are watching your waistline.) This applies particularly to meat, whole milk, and most cheeses, as these foods are major sources of fat and hence of calories. In fact, about 40 percent of the total fat intake of adults usually comes from meats and 20 percent from whole milk products. With children, these percentages are reversed. You may also want to choose relatively low-calorie selections within each group, e.g., baked potato rather than french fries. Servings of fruits and vegetables can be large because they are mostly water, but don't load those vegetables with high-calorie butter or margarine, or the fruits with excess sugar!

RECOMMENDED DIETARY ALLOWANCES

Until the end of the 1950s, nutrient-value designations known as Minimum Daily Requirements (MDR's) were used extensively in dietary recommendations and surveys. The system had certain drawbacks, however, in that it didn't take into account differences in sex and age groups, and could not satisfactorily assess the needs of large segments of the population.

The MDR's have been replaced by a more flexible and meaningful set of standards, the U.S. Recommended Daily Allowances, or USRDA's. These standards were devised by the Food and Drug Administration and are used for nutrition labeling. Unlike the old MDR's, these standards are not minimum requirements, but recommendations that incorporate a substantial margin of safety.

The USRDA's are based on another set of standards called the RDA's, or Recommended Dietary Allowances, which are set by the Food and Nutrition Board of the National Academy of Sciences. They were first developed in 1943 and have been revised at five-year intervals, most recently in 1980. The board defines the RDA's as "the levels of intake of essential nutrients considered, in the judgment of the Food and Nutrition Board on the basis of available knowledge, to be adequate to meet the known nutritional needs of practically all healthy persons."

Why are there two sets of standards, the RDA's and USRDA's? This is necessary because there are different RDA's for many different sex-age groups. This is very useful for nutrition scientists and those who counsel individuals about nutrition, but it is not useful for nutrition labeling, because there isn't room on the label to take into account all of these sex-age groups. Therefore, the USRDA was created for labeling purposes in 1974. These labeling standards are derived from the more extensive RDA's in a very simple way; the USRDA for a particular nutrient is equal to the *highest* RDA for any of the sex-age groups. This is usually the RDA that applies to teenage boys.

Only standard textbooks of nutrition published in 1980 or later would contain the 1980 RDA values and provide a full discussion of them.

Variety

Variety in the diet is important for good nutrition. Most guides for nutritious diets, such as the Basic Four Food Groups, are designed to ensure adequate intake of certain key nutrients, but this same variety helps to ensure adequate intake of all other nutrients, except the mineral fluoride. (Hence, the vital importance of fluoridation of drinking water if you happen to live in an area where the supply is low in fluoride, as many are.)

As we have mentioned, food is a very personal matter. Its enjoyment is frequently as dependent on method of preparation as on the food itself. Zucchini, for instance, may be disliked when served plain (boiled or braised) but consumed with gusto when grated into a casserole with cheese and egg. On the other hand, it may be that no one in the family exactly welcomes the presence of food such as brussels sprouts at the table, in whatever manner it may be disguised. If that is the case, there is no point in suffering with it. Your nutritional status will be little affected either way, assuming your diet includes reasonable variety otherwise.* Variety is the keystone to good nutrition, variety not only among the Basic Four Food Groups but also within each group.

Not only personal preferences but life-style, too, often affects what one eats. People with full-time jobs usually eat out more than others, and they make greater use of convenience foods. At the same time, they often wonder uncomfortably whether their own or their family's nutrition is suffering because of these eating habits. There is little reason to worry.

FAST FOOD

The alleged nutritional shortcomings of "fast food" have been well publicized by critics of our typical American eating habits. The "theory," of course, is that anyone who frequents the hamburger circuit is about to shrivel up from malnutrition and requires immediate dietary supplements.

Nutritionists have long known this was nonsense and, during the past few years, have conducted numerous studies that show it *is* nonsense. Certain independent groups, such as Consumers' Union, have performed additional nutritional analyses. The result: Among the better-known restaurant chains, a typical meal—for example, a "Big Mac" or "Whopper" or "Big Shef" or the equivalent, plus french fries and a "shake"—provides close to one-third of the average person's daily nutritional needs. It may come as a surprise that such a meal fulfills about 85 percent of a woman's RDA for protein. A meal consisting of such fare as

* We are reminded here of a "Tennessee Tuxedo" cartoon skit on television in which a modern-day Queen of Hearts had just whipped up a batch of turnip tarts from a recipe in her "health-food cookbook." The tarts were, of course, soon stolen by the knave who, after one taste, promptly returned them. But Bullwinkle, in the guise of the King of Hearts, insisted that punishment was in order: "You took them," he told the knave. "You *eat* them!"

Kentucky Fried Chicken or Pizza Hut's "Supreme" special far exceeds the daily protein requirements for anyone of any age.

The only nutritional drawback of most fast-food meals is that almost all of them are too low in vitamins A and C. (Pizza, although it contains tomato, contains little vitamin C, probably because the vitamin is largely destroyed by the high temperatures used in baking.)

Fast foods have these nutritional limitations simply because the menus of fast-food restaurants include only a small number of items. Foods that are good sources of these nutrients aren't part of the usual fast-food menu. So fast-food fans should be sure to include a wide variety of other foods in their total daily diets.

There are a couple of other precautions, but they lie in the opposite direction from the "too little" concept. One is that most fast-food emporiums tend to be overgenerous in their use of salt. If you are a regular customer and especially if you have high blood pressure, we suggest you minimize the use of salt at other meals.

Another potential problem with fast foods is their calorie count. That typical meal of a deluxe burger, fries, and shake totals up to nearly 1,200 calories. (There are slight differences among the various restaurant chains, but this figure represents a pretty fair average.) However, it is possible to choose meals at fast-food restaurants that are much lower in calories. For instance, a regular (small-size) hamburger, with its roll, plus a diet soda or a cup of black coffee adds up to only 270 calories—an amount that can be incorporated into most weight-reducing diet plans. And many fast-food places now have a salad bar, which is where you will find the vitamin A and C and lots of fiber. "Fast food" is actually a misnomer. We should speak of "fast-food service." It's the style of service, not the food that's special.

And while we're on the subject of fast meals, some readers may feel concerned about the nutritional value of "TV dinners," and similar frozen foods. While not always as flavorful, for the most part, frozen foods are very nearly as nutritious as their fresh counterparts; some are even more so if they have been fortified. Nutrients will eventually deteriorate under storage, however, the length of time varying with the type of food.

Menu Planning

Below, we have drawn up a rough general outline for distributing the Basic Four requirements throughout the day. It is assumed that these suggestions will be altered to suit individual tastes and life-styles.

Of course, you can certainly plan a nutritious diet that doesn't follow this menu plan. If you want to divide your food into five meals per day rather than three, if you want to have spaghetti for breakfast, or if you want to have your orange juice as a snack rather than as part of your morning meal, that's fine. A balanced diet can be arranged in many ways. This plan is just one simple program for getting those Basic Four Food Groups into your daily eating habits.

The possibilities for modification are endless. The point is that you attempt to include all of the needed foods at some time during every day. Our guidelines are intended only to provide a starting point for the many people who want some advice about meal planning.

Tips for Best Nutrition

We include here a few suggestions for getting these nutrients onto the table, rather than down the kitchen sink or into the garbage can.

(1) In general, nutrient levels are highest when foods are freshest. That is why commercially frozen or canned foods are equal to or even superior to home-canned or fresh foods. The fresh foods we buy in stores are not always as fresh as we think. Commercially canned or frozen foods, on the other hand, are

Suggested Daily Menu Plan

Breakfast: Fruit or juice (This should be citrus or other vitamin C-rich
food unless included elsewhere during the day.)
Cereal with milk (Or egg, toast, and milk)
Toast, if desired

Lunch: Sandwich } Or salad and bread
Fruit
Milk

Dinner: Meat, or other high-protein food
2 vegetables (Or 1 vegetable and 1 fruit)
(Include a dark green leafy vegetable or other good source of
vitamin A at least 3 times a week.)
Bread (Or rice, macaroni, etc.)
Milk (And/or pudding, ice cream, or similar milk dessert)

Add additional foods as desired to fulfill the day's calorie requirements.

"scientifically" harvested at the peak of nutritive quality. Always try to use fresh produce at its peak of ripeness, and don't overcook it.

(2) Cook vegetables in the least possible amount of water (just enough to prevent scorching), a procedure known as "short" cooking. Use cookware with tight-fitting lids.

(3) Remember that the darker portions of green vegetables have a higher nutrient content. The dark outer leaves of lettuce, for instance, may be tougher, but they are also more nutritious.

(4) Prolonged storage of frozen foods, particularly if they contain some fat, should be avoided, as off-flavors develop and there may be some loss of nutrients.

(5) Whipped potatoes and boiled peeled potatoes lose much of their vitamin C. The vitamin content is highest when they are baked or boiled with their jackets on. Some "instant" potatoes have vitamin C added. Read the label.

(6) Do not store for more than a few days partly used fruit or juice, particularly the citrus variety, for vitamin C is destroyed by exposure to air, as well as by cooking. When you do store it, or other leftovers, until the next day, do so in a covered container in the refrigerator.

(7) Drain meat and fried foods to remove some of the fat before serving. The extra fat is not needed in the usual diet and contributes extra calories that most of us don't need.

(8) Keep canned foods cool, but not below freezing.

(9) Keep frozen foods *very* cold, preferably no higher than zero degrees Fahrenheit.

Nutrition Education

Almost everyone at some point in his or her life has been introduced to the Basic Four (or the Basic Seven, or even the Basic Eleven, depending on to which generation the subject belongs). But as with so much "textbook learning," much of the information has been promptly forgotten. Even when it is retained, surveys show that many people simply never learned how to apply their knowledge to real-life eating habits. Also, classroom nutrition education has tended to be a bit dull. For some students, particularly those who belong to ethnic groups whose eating patterns do not mesh well with the Basic Four concept, it has also been confusing rather than helpful.

Youngsters may also be exposed to nutrition misinformation in school. Teachers are no more immune to the current abundance of dietary nonsense than the rest of the population, and in the experience of one of us (FJS), coaches and trainers from high school to professional levels are at the top of the totem pole when it comes to nutrition nonsense! Community groups may also introduce unsound ideas into the schools. For instance, in some areas parents' organizations have pressured local school systems to alter the school lunch program to conform to the Feingold diet or to include only "natural" foods.

There is plenty of room for improvement in the teaching of nutrition in all schools—elementary through graduate level. But it is equally important to realize that most nutrition education, like most sex education, does not occur in the classroom. Just as in the case of sex, much of what young people learn about nutrition "on the streets" is distorted or false. Young people are exposed to food fads at least as often as their elders, and they are less prepared to distinguish sound ideas from unsound ones.

Teenage girls are expecially likely to turn to unhealthful fad weight-reducing diets.

Classroom nutrition education would be improved if some time were devoted to combating current misinformation, as well as to presenting basic nutrition principles. This, of course, assumes that the teachers know the difference and from our experience, many of them don't.

Conclusion

Good eating is important for good health. And good eating is best promoted by selecting a wide variety of foods that you like from the Basic Four Food Groups every day; eating is not only a necessity, it is one of the real pleasures of life.

The end result is twofold: Physiologically, the body's requirement for the some fifty or so known nutrients is fulfilled; and psychologically, the body is treated to an assortment of other values such as taste, smell, color, texture, and temperature.

As we have stated, eating is one of the greatest pleasures of life. We want you to enjoy it to its fullest. But, as always, moderation is the key. Good nutrition, without excesses or deficiencies, is the primary goal.

The best diet for all—you, us, weight watchers, and exercise enthusiasts—is one that is enjoyable and that provides a variety of nutritious foods from the Basic Four Food Groups in amounts adequate to attain and maintain Desirable Body Weight. The key to successful weight control is *balance* between calories consumed as food and beverages and calories expended in living, in physical activity and in exercise. Thus the best way to make good nutrition a part of *your* everyday life is to obtain a bit of nutrition knowledge, modify your diet and exercise patterns, and make a varied, well-balanced diet and regular physical activity a part of your own individual life-style.

AFTERWORD

THE PURPOSE OF THIS BOOK HAS BEEN TWO-fold: to expose some of the misbeliefs and fallacious notions that have and still permeate the area of nutrition, and to introduce you to a common-sense, scientific approach to the subject.

At the very least, we hope you are now firmly aware that there is "another side" to the nutrition quandary ... that you will question and think about what you read and hear ... that you will not arrive at premature judgments based on too little knowledge or factual evidence. A large helping of common sense will remain one of your most useful allies.

Above all, we hope that you are pointed in the direction of better nutrition and better health.

ELIZABETH M. WHELAN is executive director of the American Council on Science and Health, a national, non-profit educational organization promoting scientifically balanced evaluations of food, chemicals, the environment, and human health. She holds a doctorate from the Harvard School of Public Health and a Master's degree in public health education from the Yale School of Medicine.

FREDRICK J. STARE is professor emeritus and founder of Harvard's Department of Nutrition. He is also co-founder and chairman, Board of Directors, of the American Council on Science and Health. He holds a Ph.D. from the University of Wisconsin, and an M.D. from the University of Chicago.

Both Drs. Elizabeth Whelan and Fredrick Stare have written numerous books and articles on health topics.